The compleat confectioner: or, the whole art of confectionary made plain and easy: ... By H. Glasse, ... Also, the new art of brewing. By Mr. Ellis.

Hannah Glasse

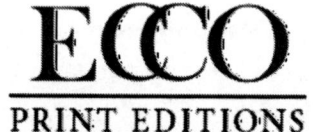

The compleat confectioner: or, the whole art of confectionary made plain and easy: ... By H. Glasse, ... Also, the new art of brewing. By Mr. Ellis.
Glasse, Hannah
ESTCID: T090908
Reproduction from British Library
Bound, and has continuous pagination with William Ellis's 'The new art of brewing ..', Dublin, 1761.
Dublin : printed by John Exshaw, 1742 [1762?].
iv,228,[16]p. ; 12°

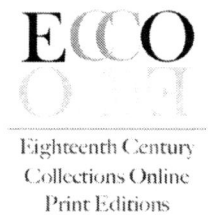

Eighteenth Century
Collections Online
Print Editions

Gale ECCO Print Editions

Relive history with *Eighteenth Century Collections Online,* now available in print for the independent historian and collector. This series includes the most significant English-language and foreign-language works printed in Great Britain during the eighteenth century, and is organized in seven different subject areas including literature and language; medicine, science, and technology; and religion and philosophy. The collection also includes thousands of important works from the Americas.

The eighteenth century has been called "The Age of Enlightenment." It was a period of rapid advance in print culture and publishing, in world exploration, and in the rapid growth of science and technology – all of which had a profound impact on the political and cultural landscape. At the end of the century the American Revolution, French Revolution and Industrial Revolution, perhaps three of the most significant events in modern history, set in motion developments that eventually dominated world political, economic, and social life.

In a groundbreaking effort, Gale initiated a revolution of its own: digitization of epic proportions to preserve these invaluable works in the largest online archive of its kind. Contributions from major world libraries constitute over 175,000 original printed works. Scanned images of the actual pages, rather than transcriptions, recreate the works *as they first appeared.*

Now for the first time, these high-quality digital scans of original works are available via print-on-demand, making them readily accessible to libraries, students, independent scholars, and readers of all ages.

For our initial release we have created seven robust collections to form one the world's most comprehensive catalogs of 18th century works.

Initial Gale ECCO Print Editions collections include:

> ### *History and Geography*
> Rich in titles on English life and social history, this collection spans the world as it was known to eighteenth-century historians and explorers. Titles include a wealth of travel accounts and diaries, histories of nations from throughout the world, and maps and charts of a world that was still being discovered. Students of the War of American Independence will find fascinating accounts from the British side of conflict.

Social Science
Delve into what it was like to live during the eighteenth century by reading the first-hand accounts of everyday people, including city dwellers and farmers, businessmen and bankers, artisans and merchants, artists and their patrons, politicians and their constituents. Original texts make the American, French, and Industrial revolutions vividly contemporary.

Medicine, Science and Technology
Medical theory and practice of the 1700s developed rapidly, as is evidenced by the extensive collection, which includes descriptions of diseases, their conditions, and treatments. Books on science and technology, agriculture, military technology, natural philosophy, even cookbooks, are all contained here.

Literature and Language
Western literary study flows out of eighteenth-century works by Alexander Pope, Daniel Defoe, Henry Fielding, Frances Burney, Denis Diderot, Johann Gottfried Herder, Johann Wolfgang von Goethe, and others. Experience the birth of the modern novel, or compare the development of language using dictionaries and grammar discourses.

Religion and Philosophy
The Age of Enlightenment profoundly enriched religious and philosophical understanding and continues to influence present-day thinking. Works collected here include masterpieces by David Hume, Immanuel Kant, and Jean-Jacques Rousseau, as well as religious sermons and moral debates on the issues of the day, such as the slave trade. The Age of Reason saw conflict between Protestantism and Catholicism transformed into one between faith and logic -- a debate that continues in the twenty-first century.

Law and Reference
This collection reveals the history of English common law and Empire law in a vastly changing world of British expansion. Dominating the legal field is the *Commentaries of the Law of England* by Sir William Blackstone, which first appeared in 1765. Reference works such as almanacs and catalogues continue to educate us by revealing the day-to-day workings of society.

Fine Arts
The eighteenth-century fascination with Greek and Roman antiquity followed the systematic excavation of the ruins at Pompeii and Herculaneum in southern Italy; and after 1750 a neoclassical style dominated all artistic fields. The titles here trace developments in mostly English-language works on painting, sculpture, architecture, music, theater, and other disciplines. Instructional works on musical instruments, catalogs of art objects, comic operas, and more are also included.

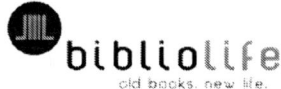

The BiblioLife Network

This project was made possible in part by the BiblioLife Network (BLN), a project aimed at addressing some of the huge challenges facing book preservationists around the world. The BLN includes libraries, library networks, archives, subject matter experts, online communities and library service providers. We believe every book ever published should be available as a high-quality print reproduction; printed on-demand anywhere in the world. This insures the ongoing accessibility of the content and helps generate sustainable revenue for the libraries and organizations that work to preserve these important materials.

The following book is in the "public domain" and represents an authentic reproduction of the text as printed by the original publisher. While we have attempted to accurately maintain the integrity of the original work, there are sometimes problems with the original work or the micro-film from which the books were digitized. This can result in minor errors in reproduction. Possible imperfections include missing and blurred pages, poor pictures, markings and other reproduction issues beyond our control. Because this work is culturally important, we have made it available as part of our commitment to protecting, preserving, and promoting the world's literature.

GUIDE TO FOLD-OUTS MAPS and OVERSIZED IMAGES

The book you are reading was digitized from microfilm captured over the past thirty to forty years. Years after the creation of the original microfilm, the book was converted to digital files and made available in an online database.

In an online database, page images do not need to conform to the size restrictions found in a printed book. When converting these images back into a printed bound book, the page sizes are standardized in ways that maintain the detail of the original. For large images, such as fold-out maps, the original page image is split into two or more pages

Guidelines used to determine how to split the page image follows:

• Some images are split vertically; large images require vertical and horizontal splits.
• For horizontal splits, the content is split left to right.
• For vertical splits, the content is split from top to bottom.
• For both vertical and horizontal splits, the image is processed from top left to bottom right.

1037 d. 29

THE
Compleat Confectioner:

OR, THE

Whole Art of Confectionary

Made PLAIN and EASY:

SHEWING,

The various Methods of PRESERVING and CANDYING, both dry and liquid, all Kinds of FRUIT, FLOWERS and HERBS, the different Ways of CLARIFYING SUGAR, and the Method of Keeping FRUIT, NUTS and FLOWERS fresh and fine all the Year round.

ALSO

DIRECTIONS for making

ROCK-WORKS and CANDIES,	STRONG CORDIAL,
BISCUITS,	SIMPLE WATERS,
RICH CAKES,	MEAD, OILS, &c.
CREAMS,	SYRUPS of all Kinds,
CUSTARDS,	MILK PUNCH, that will keep
JELLIES,	twenty Yeras
WHIP SYLLABUBS, and CHEESE-CAKES of all Sorts	KNICKNACKS and TRIFLES for DESERTS, &c
ENGLISH WINES of all Sorts	

LIKEWISE

The Art of making ARTIFICIAL FRUIT, with the Stalks in it, so as to resemble the natural Fruit.

To which are added,
Some BILLS of FARE for DESERTS for private FAMILIES.

By H GLASSE, Author of the ART of COOKERY.

ALSO,
The NEW ART OF BREWING By Mr ELLIS.

DUBLIN

Printed by JOHN EXSHAW, at the Bible in Dame-street,

MDCCXLII

TO THE

HOUSE-KEEPERS

OF

Great Britain and *Ireland*

T HERE is, perhaps, no book more wanted, than a Compleat Confectioner. Several little pieces have been written on this subject; but none on a plan extensive enough for general use. Ladies who reside chiefly in the country, where they have no opportunity of procuring things from a confectioner, must very sensibly feel the want of such a book as this, and those who have hitherto bought of the Confectioners, will soon find, that a vast expence is to be saved by the use of this book, which is compiled, partly from the manuscripts of a very old experienced housekeeper to a family of the first distinction, and partly from my own experience. I do not take on me to direct the setting out a grand desert, as that must depend on each Lady's particular fancy, but I have given some few bills of fare, for deserts in private families, where they may be at a loss to think of things in a hurry.

You

[iv]

You will also herein find, the Art of joining China-ware, so as to be fit for use in ten minutes, provided the ingredients are ready to join it with. I have said nothing on cookery, having already written fully on that subject, in a work, intituled, The Art of Cookery made Plain and Easy, which, together with this book, I flatter myself, will be sufficient to compleat the young, and unexperienced Ladies, in every branch of housekeeping.

I am, with the greatest respect, Ladies, your most obedient humble Servant,

H. GLASSE.

⁎ The Publisher of this Edition, begs Leave to mention how much he has improved it, by the addition of a great Number of Receipts in the Article of Distilling, and Family Cordials, with some of the most approved Washes and Essences now in Use, and the entire Piece, Of the new Art of Brewing and improving Malt Liquors to the greatest Advantage, including all the Improvements that have been lately made, collected from the present Practice of the best Brewers in England, and put into Order by WILLIAM ELLIS, Brewer.

THE COMPLEAT CONFECTIONER.

To clarify sugar.

BREAK into your preserving-pan the white of an egg, put in four quarts of water, beat it up to a froth with a whisk, then put in twelve pounds of sugar, mixed together, set it over the fire, and when it boils put in it a little cold water, so do for four or five times, till the scum appears thick on the top; then remove it from the fire, and let it settle; then take off the scum, and pass it through your straining-bag.

Note If the sugar doth not appear very fine, you must boil it again before you strain it, otherwise, in boiling it to a height, it will rise over the pan.

To boil sugar to the degree called smooth.

When your sugar is thus clarified, put what quantity you have occasion for over the fire, to boil smooth, which you'll prove by dipping your scummer into the sugar, and then touching it with your fore-finger and thumb; in opening them, you will see a small thread drawn betwixt, which immediately breaks and remains in a drop on your thumb; thus it is a little smoath then boiling more, it will draw into a larger string, then it is become very smooth.

The blown sugar

Boil your sugar longer than the former, and try it thus, *viz* dip in your scummer, and take it out, shaking off what sugar you can into the pan, and then blow with your mouth strongly through the holes; and if certain bubbles or bladders blow through, it is boiled to the degree called blown

The feathered sugar

It is a higher degree of boiling sugar, which is to be proved by dipping the scummer, when it hath boiled somewhat longer; shake it first over the pan, then give it a sudden flurt behind you; if it be enough, the sugar will fly off like feathers.

The crackled sugar,

Is proved by letting it boil somewhat longer, and then dipping a stick into the sugar, which immediately remove into a pot of cold water, standing by for that purpose, drawing off the sugar that cleaves to the stick, if it becomes hard, and will snap in the water, it is enough; if not, you must boil it till it comes to that degree

Note · Your water must be always very cold or it will deceive you

The carmel sugar,

Is known by boiling yet longer; and is proved by dipping a stick, as aforesaid, first in the sugar, and then in the water but this you must observe, when it comes to the carmel height, it will snap like glass the
moment

ment it touches the cold water, which is the highest and last degree of boiling sugar.

Note. Observe that your fire be not very fierce when you boil this, lest, flaming up the sides of your pan, it should cause the sugar to burn, and so discolour it.

To preserve Seville oranges liquid, as also lemons

Take the best Seville oranges and pare them very neatly, put them into salt and water for about two hours, then boil them very tender, till a pin will go into them easily, then drain them well from the water and put them into your preserving pan, putting as much clarified sugar to them as will cover them, laying a trencher or plate on them to keep them down, then set them over a fire, and by degrees heat them till they boil; let them have a quick boil, till the sugar comes all over them in a froth, then set them by till next day, when you must drain the syrup from them, and boil it till it becomes very smooth, adding some more clarified sugar; put it upon the oranges, and give them a boil, then set them by till next day, when you must do as the day before. The fourth day drain them, and strain your syrup through a bag, and boil it till it becomes very smooth; then take some other clarified sugar, boil it till it blows very strong, and take some jelly of pippins, as I shall hereafter express, with the juice of some other oranges, after they are preserved as above directed, take two pounds of clarified sugar, boil it to blow very strong; then one pint and a half of pippin jelly, and the juice of four or five oranges, boil all together; then put in the syrup that has been strained and boiled to be very smooth, and give all a boil; then put your oranges into your pots, or glasses, and fill them up with the above made jelly, when cold, cover them and set them by for use.

Note. Be sure in all your boilings to clear away the scum, otherwise you will endanger their working, and if you find they will swim above your jelly, you must bind them down with the sprig of a clean whisk.

THE COMPLEAT

To draw a jelly from pippins

Take the fairest and firmest pippins, pour them into fair water, as much as will cover them, set them over a quick fire and boil them to mash, then put them on a sieve over an earthen pan, and press out all the jelly, which jelly strain through a bag, and use as directed in the oranges before-mentioned, and such others as shall be hereafter prescribed

To make orange marmalade, also lemon

Take six oranges, grate two of the rinds of them upon a grater, then cut them all, and pick out the flesh from the skin and seeds; put to it the grated rind, and about half a pint of pippin jelly, take the same weight of sugar as you have of this meat so mingled; boil your sugar till it blows very strong, then put in the meat, and boil all very quick till it becomes a jelly, which you will find by dipping the scummer and holding it up to drain; if it be a jelly, it will break from the scummer in flakes, and if not, it will run off in little streams, when it is a good jelly, put it into your glasses or pots

Note· If you find this composition too sweet, you may, in boiling, add more juice of oranges, the different quickness they have makes it difficult to prescribe

To preserve oranges with marmalade in them, and lemons

Pare your oranges as before; make a round hole in the bottom, where the stalk grew, the bigness of a shilling, take out the meat and put them into salt and water for two or three hours, then boil them very tender and put them into a clarified sugar; give them a boil the next day, drain the syrup and boil it till it becomes smooth; put in your oranges, and give them a good boil, when a little cool, drain them, and fill them with a marmalade made as before directed,

putting

putting in the round piece you cut out, with the syrup, some other sugar, and pippin juice, make a jelly, and fill up your pots and glasses.

For variety, take three of your preserved oranges, take off the tops, cut them so as to look like little cups, and fill them with this marmalade; they both eat pretty, and make a variety.

To preserve green oranges

Take the green oranges, slit them on one side, and put them into a brine of salt water, as strong as will bear an egg, in which you must soak them at least fifteen days, then strain them and put them into fresh water, and boil them tender, then put them into fresh water again, shifting them every day for five days together, then give them another scald, and put them into a clarified sugar; then give them a boil, and set them by till next day; then boil them again; the next day add some more sugar, and give them another boil; the day after boil the syrup very smooth, pour it on them and keep them.

Note That if at any time you perceive the syrup begin to work, you must drain them and boil the syrup very smooth, and pour it on them, but if the first proves sour, you must boil it likewise. Green lemons are done after the same manner.

Note also, If the oranges are any thing large, you you must take out the meat from the in-side.

To make a compote of oranges.

Cut the rind off your oranges into ribs, leaving part of the rind on; cut them into eight parts, and throw them into boiling water, when a pin will easily go through the rind, drain and put them into as much sugar, boiled till it becomes smooth, as will cover them, give all a boil together, adding some juice of oranges to what sharpness you please; you may put a little pippin jelly into the boiling; when cold, they make pretty plates.

The Dutchess of Cleveland's receipt to preserve lemons, citrons and oranges.

Take good lemons, fair and well coloured, and scrape a little of the uppermost rind, take out the seeds, and the juice, lay them in spring water, shifting them twice a day for a day or two, then boil them, to be tender, with a pound and quarter of double-refined sugar, and a pint and three quarters of spring water, take the scum off, and put in your lemons, have ready a pint of pippin water, boil it first with half a pound of sugar, and put it to them; then boil it to a jelly, and put in the juice of your lemons, then let them boil, but a little after, and put them into your glasses, but be sure to cover them with syrup.

How to take out the seeds.

You must cut a hole in the top, but it must be a little one, and take them out with a scoop, dry them, before you put them into your syrup, with a clean cloth.

To make orange rings and faggots.

Pare your oranges as thin and as narrow as you can; put the parings into water whilst you prepare the rings, which are done by cutting the oranges, so pared, into as many rings as you please; then cut out the meat from the inside, and put the rings and faggots into boiling water, boil them till they tender, then put them into as much clarified sugar as will cover them, set them by till next day, then boil them all together, and set them by till the day after; then drain the syrup and boil it till very smooth, then return your oranges into it, and give all a boil; the next day boil the syrup till it rises up to almost the top of your pan, then return your oranges into it, give them a boil, and put them by in some pot to be candied, as hereafter mentioned, whenever you shall have occasion.

Zest of China oranges.

Pare off the outward rind of the oranges very thin, and only strew it with fine powder sugar, as much as their own moisture will take, and dry them in a hot stove.

To candy orange, lemon, and citron

Drain what quantity you will candy clean from the syrup, wash it in luke-warm water, and lay it on a sieve to drain; then take as much clarified sugar as you think will cover what you will candy, boil it till it blows very strong, then put in your rings, and boil them till it blows again; then take it from the fire, let it cool a little, and, with the back of a spoon, rub the sugar against the inside of your pan, till you see the sugar becomes white; then, with a fork, take out the rings one by one, and lay them on a wire grate to drain; then put in your faggots, and boil them as before directed; then rub the sugar, and take them up in bunches, having somebody to cut them with a pair of scissars to what bigness you please, laying them on your wire to drain.

Note Thus you may candy all sorts of oranges, lemon peels, or chips; lemon rings and faggots are done the same way, with this distinction only, that the lemons ought to be pared twice over, that the ring may be the whiter; so will you have two sorts of faggots, but you must be sure to keep the outward rind from the other, otherwise it will discolour them.

To make orange cakes

Take six Seville oranges, grate the rinds of two of them, then cut off the rinds of all six to the juice, and boil them in water till very tender; then squeeze out all the water you can, and beat them to a paste in a marble mortar; rub it through a hair sieve, and what will not easily rub through, must be beaten again till it will, cut to pieces the insides of your oranges, and rub as much of them through as you possibly can, then boil about six or eight pippins in as much water as will almost cover them, boil them to a paste, and rub it through a sieve to the rest, put all into a pan together, and give them a thorough heat till they are well mingled, then, to every pound of this paste, take one pound and a quarter of loaf sugar, clarify the sugar, and boil it to the crick, put in your paste and the grated peel, and stir it all together, over a low fire, till it is well mixed, and the sugar all melted, then, with a spoon, fill your round tin moulds, and set them in a warm stove to dry, when dry on the tops, turn them on sieves to dry on the other side; and when quite dry box them up

Lemon cakes.

Take six thick rined lemons, grate two of them, then pare off all the yellow peel, and strip the white to the juice, which white boil till tender, and make a paste exactly as above

To preserve white citrons

Cut your white citrons into what sized pieces you please, put them into water and salt for four or five hours, then wash them in fair water, and boil them till tender, drain them, and put them into as much clarified sugar as will cover them, and set them by till next day; then drain the syrup, and boil it a little smooth, when cool, put in your citrons, the next day boil your syrup quite smooth, and pour on your citrons, the day after boil all together, and put it into a pot to be candied, or put it into jellies, or compose it as you please

You may make fine citron of green melons

Cut them all long ways into quarters; scrape out the seeds and inside, and preserve and candy the same above, only with this difference, boil them three times up in the syrup

Note. You must look over these fruits kept in syrup, and if you perceive any froth on them, you must give them a boil; and if they should become very frothy and sour, you must first boil the syrup, and then all together.

To make orange clear cakes

Take the best pippins, pare them into as much water as will cover them, and boil them to a mash, then press out the jelly upon a sieve, and strain it thro' a bag, adding juice of oranges to give it an agreeable taste, to every pound of jelly take one pound and a quarter of loaf sugar, boil it till it cracks, and then put in the jelly and the rind of a grated orange or two, stir it up gently over a slow fire, till all is incorporated together; then take it off, and fill your clear cake glasses; what scum arises on the top, you must carefully take off before they are cold; then put them into a stove, and when you find them begin to crust upon the upper side, turn them out upon squares of glasses and put them to dry again, when they begin to have a tender candy, cut them into quarters or what pieces you please, and let them dry till hard, then turn them on sieves, and, when thorough dry, put them in your boxes.

Note As they begin to sweat in the box, you must shift them from time to time, and it will be requisite to put no more than one row in a box, at the beginning, till they do not sweat Lemon colour cakes are made with lemons as these.

To make orange flower paste

Boil one pound of the leaves of orange flowers very tender, then take two pounds and two ounces of double-refined sugar in fine powder, and when you have bruised the flowers to a pulp, stir in the sugar by degrees, over a slow fire, till all is in and well melted, then make little drops and dry them.

To preserve orange flowers.

Take the orange flowers just as they begin to open, put them into boiling water, and let them boil very quick till they are tender, putting in a little juice of lemon, as they boil, to keep them white; then drain them, and dry them carefully between two napkins; then put them into clarified sugar, as much as will cover them, the next day drain the syrup, and boil it a little smooth, when almost co'd, pour it on the flowers, and the next day you may drain them and lay them out to dry, dusting them a very little

To put them in jelly.

After they are preserved, as before directed, you must clarify a little more sugar, with orange flower water, and make a jelly of codlins, which, when ready, put in the flowers, syrup, and all, give them a boil, scum them, and put them into your glasses or pots

To make orange flower cakes.

Take four ounces of the leaves of orange flowers, put them into fair water for about an hour, then drain them and put them between two napkins, and, with a rolling-pin, roll them till they are bruised, then have ready boiled, one pound of double-refined sugar, to a bloom degree, put in the flowers, and boil it till it comes to the same degree again, then remove it from the fire, and let it cool a little; then, with a spoon, grind the sugar to the bottom or sides of the pan, and when it becomes white, pour it into little papers or cards made in the form of a dripping-pan, and, when quite cold, take them out of the pans, and dry them a little in a stove

To make pomegranate clear cakes

Draw your jelly as for the orange clear cakes, then boil it in the juice of two or three pomegranate seeds,
and

and all with the juice of an orange and lemon, the rind of each grated in; then strain it through a bag, and to every pound of jelly, put one pound and a quarter, boiled till it cracks, to help the colour to a fine red, put in a spoonful of cochineal, prepared as hereafter directed, and then fill your glasses, and order them as oranges

To preserve cochineal

Take one ounce of cochineal and beat it to a fine powder; then boil it in three quarters of a pint of water to the consumption of half, then beat half an ounce of roach alum, and half an ounce of cream of tartar, very fine, and put them to the cochineal, boil them all together a little while, and strain it through a fine bag, which put into a phial and keep for use

Note · If an ounce of loaf sugar be boiled in with it, it will keep from moulding what you do not use immediately

To make pippin knots

Take your pippins and weigh them, then put them into your preserving-pan, to every pound put four ounces of sugar, and as much water as will scarce cover them, boil them to a pulp, and then pulp them through a sieve, then, to every pound of the apples weighed, take one pound of sugar clarified; boil it till it almost cracks, then put in the paste, and mix it well over a slow fire; then take it off, and pour it on flat pewter plates, or the bottoms of dishes, to the thickness of two crowns, and set them in the stove for three or four hours, then cut it into narrow slips, and turn it up into knots to what shape or size you please, put them into the stove to dry, dusting them a little; turn them, and dry them on the other side, and, when thorough dry, put them into your box

Note You may make them red, by adding a little cochineal, or green, by putting a little of the following colour

To prepare a green colour

Take gambouge one quarter of an ounce, of indico and blue the same quantity; beat them very fine in a brass mortar, and mix with it a spoonful of water, so you will have a fine green

To preserve golden pippins in jelly

Pare your pippins from all spots, and, with a narrow-pointed knife, make a hole quite through them, then boil them in fair water about a quarter of an hour, drain them, and take as much sugar as will cover them, boil it till it blows very strong, then put in your pippins, and give them a good boil, let them cool a little, and give them another, then if you have, for example, a dozen of pippins, take a pound of sugar, and boil it till it blows very strong, then put in half a pint of pippin jelly, and the juice of three or four lemons, boil all together, and put to the golden pippins; give them all a boil, scum them, and put them into glasses or pots

To preserve pippins for present eating

Pare them very thin and put them into a clean stewpan, saucepan, or preserving-pan, according to the quantity you want, but scoop out the cores, and into every pippin put two or three long narrow bits of lemon peel, take the parings, boil them in water enough to cover the pippins, strain it, and make it as sweet as syrup, pour it on your pippins, and stew them til they are quite tender; they make a pretty plate

To dry golden pippins

Pare your pippins, and make a hole in them as above, then weigh them and boil them till tender, take them out of the water, and to every pound of pippins take a pound and a half of loaf sugar, and boil it till it blows very strong,
then

then put in the fruit, and boil it very quick till the sugar flows all over the pan, let them settle, cool them, scum them, and set them by till the next day, then drain them and lay them out to dry, dusting them with fine sugar before you put them into the stove, the next day turn them and dust them again; when dry, pack them up

You may dry them in slices, or quarters, after the same manner

To green codlins

Take your codlins, and coddle them gently, close covered, then peel your codlins, and put them into cold water, setting them over a slow fire till they are green, close covered ; they will be two or three hours doing

To dry apples or pears

First boil them in new ale worth, on a slow fire, for a quarter of an hour, then take them out and press them flat, and dry them in your oven, or stove ; put them up in papers, in a box, and they will keep all the year

To make black caps of apples.

Pare them, lay them in your pan, strew a few cloves over them, a little lemon peel cut very small, and two or three blades of cinnamon, with some coarse sugar; cover the pan with brown paper, set them in an oven with the bread, and let them stand till the oven is cold

To make a compote of bonchretien pears.

Pare your fruit, and cut them into slices; scald them a little, squeezing some juice of lemon on them, in the scalding, to keep them white ; then drain them, and put as much clarified sugar as will just cover them; give them a boil, and then squeeze the juice of an orange

range or lemon, which you best approve of, and serve them to table when cold

A compote of baked wardens

Bake your wardens in an earthen pot, with a little claret, some spice, lemon peel, and sugar; when you use them, peel off the skin and dress them in plates, either whole or in halves; then make a jelly of pippins, sharpened well with the juice of lemons, and pour it upon them; when cold, break the jelly with a spoon, and it will look very agreeable upon the red pears

To stew pears purple

First pare your pears, then cut them in two, or whole; lay them in a stew-pan, and boil the parings in water, just sufficient to cover them; strain it off, and make it as sweet as syrup; pour it over your pears, and lay a pewter plate on them, putting on the cover of the stew-pan close, and let them stew over a slow fire for half an hour, or till they are quite tender, and they will be a fine purple

To rock candy violets.

Pick the leaves off the violets, then boil some of the finest sugar till it blows very strong, which pour into your candying pan, being made of tin in the form of a dripping-pan, about three inches deep, then strew the leaves of the flowers as thick on the top as you can, and put it into a hot stove for eight or ten days; when you see it is hard candied, break a hole in one corner of it, and drain all the syrup that will run from it, break it out, and lay it on heaps on plates to dry in the stove

To candy violets whole

Take the double violets, and pick off the green stalks, then boil some sugar till it blows very strong,
then

then throw in the violets, and boil it till it blows again, then, with a spoon, rub the sugar against the sides of the pan, till white; then stir all till the sugar leaves them, and then sift and dry them

Note: Jonquils are done the same way.

To preserve angelica in knots.

Take young and thick stalks of angelica, cut them into lengths of about a quarter of a yard, and scald them, then put them into water, strip off the skins, and cut them into narrow slips; lay them on your preserving pan, and put to them a thin sugar, that is, to one part sugar, as clarified, and one part water, then set it over the fire, let it boil, and set it by till next day, then turn it in the pan, give it another boil, and the day after drain it and boil the sugar till it is a little smooth; pour it on your angelica, and if it be a good green boil it no more, if not, heat it again, and the day following boil the sugar till it is very smooth, and pour it upon your angelica, the next day boil your syrup till it rises to the top of your pan, and put your angelica into your pan; pour your syrup upon it, and keep it for use.

To dry it.

Drain what quantity you will from the syrup, and boil as much sugar as will cover it, till it blows, put in your angelica, and give it a boil till it blows again; then cold, drain it, tie it in knots, and put it into a warm stove to dry, first dusting it a little; when dry on one side, turn it to dry on the other, and then pack it up

To preserve angelica in sticks.

Angelica, not altogether so young as the other, cut into short pieces, about half a quarter of a yard, or less, scald it a little, then drain it, and put it into a thin sugar as before, boil it a little the next day, turn

turn it in the pan the bottom upwards and boil it, and then finish it as the other for knots

Note When you will candy it, you must drain it from the syrup, wash it, and candy it as the orange and lemon

Angelica paste

Take the youngest and most pithy angelica you can get, boil it very tender, and drain and press out all the water you possibly can; then beat it in a mortar to as fine a paste as may be, and rub it through a sieve, next day dry it over a fire, and, to every pound of this paste, take one pound of fine sugar in fine powder; when your paste is hot, put in the sugar, stirring it over a gentle fire till it is well incorporated; when so done, drop it on plates, long or round, as you think proper, dust it a little, and put it into the stove to dry.

To preserve ringoe root

Take your ringoe roots, and parboil them reasonably tender, then pick and peel them, wash them very clean, dry them with a cloth, and put in as much clarified sugar as will cover them, boil them leisurely in a great silver bason that is deep, set on a chafing dish of coals, till you see the rolls look clear and your syrup something thick, betwixt hot and cold, and put them up

To preserve sweet-marjoram.

Take the white of an egg, beat it very well, and take double refined sugar, beaten very fine and sifted; then take the marjoram, and rub it on a glass that is clear, and lay it in form of the glass, so do it with your egg, then sect it with your sugar on it, and lay it on papers to dry

To preserve quinces white

Pare and core the quinces; to every pound of sugar and quinces, put in a pint of water, boil them together as fast as you can, uncovered. The same way you may preserve pippins white.

To preserve quinces white or red.

Core and pare your quinces; those which you would have white, put into a pail of water for two or three hours; then take as much sugar as they weigh, and add as much water as will make a syrup to cover them, boil the syrup a little, then put in the quinces, and let them boil as fast as you can till they are very tender and clear; afterwards take them out, and boil the syrup a little higher alone, and when it is cold put the quinces up in pots; if you would have them red, put them raw into sugar and let them boil gently, being close covered, till they are red; you must not put them into cold water.

The jelly

Take a quantity of spring water, and put into it as many quinces, thin sliced, and cores and parings, as will conveniently boil to be tender, also a large handful of hartshorn, boil it very fast, keeping it stirring; when it is strong enough tasted, rub it through a jelly bag this is best when it looks pure white, let your hartshorn be boiled first, add this to your syrup, and boil it altogether

To preserve apricots green

Take the apricots when about to stone, before it becomes too hard for a pin easily to pass through; pare them in ribs very neatly, because every stroke with the knife will be seen, then put them into fair water as you pare them, and boil them till tender enough to slip easily from your pin, drain them,

them, and put them into a thin sugar, that is to say, one part sugar clarified, and one part water, boil them a little, and set them by till next day, then give them another boil, and the day after drain them, boil your syrup a little smooth, and put it upon them without boiling your fruit, let them remain in the syrup four or five days, then boil some more sugar till it blows hard, and add it to them, give all a boil and let them lie till the day following, then drain them from the syrup, and lay them out to dry, dusting them with a little fine sugar before you put them into the stove

To put them up in jelly

You must keep them in the syrup till codlins are pretty well grown, taking care to visit them sometimes that they do not sour, which, if they do, the syrup will be lost, by reason it will become muddy, and then you will be obliged to make your jelly with all fresh sugar, which will be too sweet, but when codlins are of an indifferent bigness, draw a jelly from them as from pippins, as you are directed in the foregoing receipts, then drain the apricots from the syrup, boil it and strain it through your straining bags, then boil some sugar, proportionably to the quantity of apricots you design to put up, till it blows, then put in the jelly, and boil it a little with the sugar, then put in the syrup and the apricots, and give them all a boil together till you find the syrup will be a jelly; then remove them from the fire, scum them well, and put them into your pots or glasses, observing, as they cool, if they be regular in the glasses, to sink and disperse them to a proper distance, and, when quite cold, to cover them up

To preserve apricots whole

Take the apricots when full grown, pare them, and take out their stones; then have ready a pan of boiling water, throw them into it, and scald them till they rise to the top of the water, take them out carefully

fully with your scummer, and lay them on a sieve to drain, then lay them in your preserving pan, and lay over them as much sugar, boiled to blow, as will cover them; give them a boil round, by setting the pan half on the fire, and turning it about as it boils; then set it full on the fire, and let it have a covered boiling, then let them settle a quarter of an hour and pick those that look clear to one side, and those that do not, to the other, boil that side that is not clear, till they become clear, and, as they do so, pick them away, left they boil to a paste; when you see they look all alike, give them a covered boiling, scum them, and set them by, the next day, boil a little more sugar to blow very strong, put it to the apricots, and give them a very good boil; scum and cover them with paper, and put them in a stove for two days; then drain them and lay them out to dry, first dusting the plates you lay them on, and then the apricots extraordinary well, blowing off what sugar lies white upon them; put them into a very warm stove to dry, and when dry, on one side, turn and dust them again; when quite dry, pack them up.

Note. In the turning them, you must take care there be no little bladders in them; if there be, you must prick them with the point of a penknife, and squeeze them out, otherwise they will blow and sour.

To preserve apricot chips.

Split the apricots, and then take out the stones; pare them, and turn them round with your knife; put them into your pan without scalding, and put as much sugar, boiled very smooth, as will cover them; then manage them on the fire as the whole apricots, scum them, and set them in the stove, the next day boil some more sugar, very strong, drain the syrup from the apricots boil it very smooth, put it to the fresh sugar, and give it a boil; then put in the apricots, boil them first round, and then let them have a covered boil, scum them and cover them with paper, then put them into the stove

for

for two or three days, drain them, and lay them out to dry, first dusting them

To preserve apricots in jellies.

Pare and stone your apricots, then scald them a little, then lay them in your pan, and put as much clarified sugar to them as will cover them, the next day drain the syrup, and boil it smooth, then slip in your apricots, and boil as before; the next day make a jelly with codlins, boiling some apricots among them to give a better taste, when you have boiled the jelly to its proper height, put in the apricots with their syrop, and boil all together, when enough, scum them well, and put them into your glasses

To make apricot paste

Boil some apricots that are full ripe to a pulp, and rub the fine of it through a sieve; to every pound of pulp, take one pound two ounces of fine sugar, beaten to a very fine powder, heat well your paste, and by degrees put in your sugar, when all is in, give it a thorough heat over the fire, taking care not to let it boil, then take it off, and scrape it all to one side of the pan; let it cool a little, then lay it out on plates in what form you please; then dust them, and put them into the stove to dry

To make apricot clear cakes

First draw a jelly from codlins, and, in that jelly boil some very ripe apricots, and press them upon a sieve over an earthen pan, then strain it through your jelly bag, and to every pound of jelly take the like quantity of fine loaf sugar, which clarify and boil till it cracks, then put in the jelly, mix it well, and give it a heat on the fire, scum it and fill your glasses, in drying them order them as before directed

To make apricot jam

Pare the apricots; take out the stones, break them, take out the kernels and blanch them, then, to every pound of apricots boil one pound of sugar, till it blows very strong, then put in the apricots, and boil them very brisk, till they are all broke, then take them off, bruise them well, put in the kernels, and stir them all together over the fire; then fill your pots or glasses with them

To preserve nectarines

Split the nectarines, and take out the stones, then put them into a clarified sugar, and boil them round till they have well taken sugar, take off the scum, cover them with a paper, and set them by, the next day boil a little more sugar, till it blows very strong, put it to the nectarines, and give them a good boil; take off the scum, cover them and put them into the stove, the next day drain them, and lay them out to dry first dusting them a little, then put them into the stove again.

To preserve peaches whole

Take the Newington peach, when full ripe, split it and take out the stone; then have ready a pan of boiling water, drop in the peaches, and let them have a few moments scalding; take them out, and put them into as much sugar, only clarified, as will cover them; give them a boil round, then scum them and set them by till the next day; then boil some more sugar to blow very strong, which sugar put to the peaches and give them a good boil, scum them and set them by till the day following, then give them another good boil, scum them and put them into a warm stove for the space of two days, then drain them and lay them out, one half over the other, dust them and put them into the stove; the next day turn them and dust them, and, when thorough dry, pack them up for use

How

How to preserve peach chips.

Pare your peaches and take out the stones, then cut them into very thin slices, not thicker than the blade of a knife, then, to every pound of chips take one pound and a half of sugar, boiled to blow very strong; throw in the chips, give them a good boil and let them settle a little; take off the scum, let them stand a quarter of an hour, and then give them another good boil, and let them settle as before; then take off the scum, cover them and set them by, and the next day drain them and lay them out, bit by bit; dust them and dry them in a warm stove; when dry on one side, take them from the plate with a knife and turn them on a sieve, and then again, if they are not pretty dry, which they generally are

How to put them in jelly

Draw a jelly from codlins, and when they are boiled enough to take as much jelly as sugar, boil the sugar to blow very strong; then put in the jelly, give it a boil, and put it to the chips, give all a boil scum them, and put them into your glasses.

How to preserve peaches in brandy

First preserve your peaches whole, with their weight of sugar, do not scald them in water, but boil them into the syrup three times; lay your peaches in a large deep glass for the purpose, take the syrup and pour it over them, with an equal quantity of brandy, cover them close and keep them for use.

Nectarines do the same way

To preserve violet plumbs.

Violet plumbs are a long time yellow, and are ripe in the month of June; they are preserved as follow, put them into clarified sugar, just enough to cover them,

them, and boil them pretty quick, the next day boil them again as before; the day after drain them and take away their skins, which you will find all flown off, then put them into sugar boiled till it blows a little, and give them a boil; the day following boil some more sugar till it blows a little, and give them another boil, the next day boil some more sugar to blow very strong, put it to the plumbs in the syrup, boil them a little, scum them, the next day drain them, and lay them out to dry, observing to dust them before you put them into the stove.

How to preserve green amber plumbs.

Take the green amber-plumbs when full grown, prick them in two or three places, and put them into cold water; set them over the fire to scald, in which you must be very careful not to let the water be too hot, lest you hurt them, when they are very tender, put them into a very thin sugar, that is to say, one part sugar and two parts water; give them a little warm in this sugar, cover them, and the next day give them another warm; the third day drain them, and boil the syrup, adding a little more sugar; then put the syrup to the plumbs, and give them a boil, and the day after boil the syrup till very smooth; then put it to the plumbs, cover them, and put them into the stove, the next day boil some more sugar to blow very strong, put it to the fruit, give all a boil, and put them into the stove for two days, then drain them, and lay them out to dry, first dusting them very well; manage them in the drying as other fruit

To preserve fruit green

Take pippins, apricots, pear plumbs or peaches, while they are green, and put them in a preserving-pan, or stew-pan; cover them with vine leaves, and then with fine clear spring water, put on the cover of the pan, set them over a clear fire, when they begin to simmer take them off, and carefully with your
slice

slice take them out, peel and preserve them as you do other fruit.

To preserve green orange plumbs.

Take the green orange plumbs, full grown, before they turn, prick them with a fine bodkin, as thick all over as you possibly can; put them into cold water, as you prick them, and when all are done, set them over a very slow fire and scald them with the utmost care you can, nothing being so subject to break, and if the skin flies they are worth nothing, when they are tender, take them off the fire, and set them by in the same water for two or three days; when they become sour, and begin to fret on the top of the water, be careful to drain them very well, and put them in single rows in your preserving-pan; put to them as much thin sugar as will cover them, that is to say, one part sugar and two parts water; set them over the fire, and by degrees warm them, till you perceive the sourness to be gone, and the plumbs are sunk to the bottom; then set them by, and the next day throw away that syrup, and put to them a fresh sugar of one part sugar and one part water, in this sugar give them several heats, but not to boil, lest you hurt them; cover them and set them in a warm stove, that they may suck in what sugar they can; the next day drain the sugar, and boil it till it becomes smooth, adding some more fresh sugar; pour this sugar on them, return them into the stove, and the day after boil the sugar to become very smooth, pour it upon the plumbs, and give all a gentle boil, scum it and put them into the stove; the day following drain them out of the syrup, and boil some fresh sugar, as much as you judge will cover them, very smooth, put it to your plumbs, and give all a very good covered boiling; then take off the scum, cover them, and let them stand in the stove two days, then drain and lay them out to dry, dusting them very well

To preserve the green Mogul plumb

Take this plumb when just upon turning ripe, prick with a penknife, to the very stone on that side where the cleft is, and put them into cold water as you do them, then set them over a very slow fire to scald, and when they are become very tender, take them carefully out of the water and put them into a thin sugar, that is, half sugar and half water; warm them gently, cover them, and set them by, the next day, give them another warm and set them by; the day following drain the syrup and boil it smooth, adding to it a little fresh sugar, and give them a gentle boil, the day after boil the sugar very smooth, pour it upon them, and set them in the stove for two days; drain them, and boil a fresh sugar to be very smooth, or just to blow a little, and put it to your plumbs, give them a good covered boiling, scum them, and put them into a stove for two days, drain them, and lay them out to dry, dusting them very well

To preserve the green admirable plumb

This is a little round plumb, about the size of a damson. it leaves the stone when ripe, is somewhat inclining to a yellow in colour, and very well deserves its name, being the finest green when done, and with a tenth part of the trouble and charge, as you will find by the receipt

Take this plumb when full grown, and just upon the turn; prick them with a penknife in two or three places, and scald them by degrees till the water becomes very hot, for they will even bear boiling, continue them in the water till they become green, then drain them and put them into a clarified sugar; boil them very well, and let them settle a little, then give them another boil, if you perceive they shrink and take not the sugar in very well; prick them with a fork all over, as they lie in the pan, and give them another boil, scum them, and set them by, the next day boil some other sugar, till it blows, and put it to them; give them another boil, set them in the stove for one night; and the next day drain them and lay them out, first dusting them.

To preserve yellow amber plumbs

Take these plumbs when full ripe, put them into your preserving-pan, and put to them as much sugar as will cover them; give them a very good boil, let them settle a little, and give them another boil three or four times round, scum them, and the next day drain them from the syrup, return them again into the pan, boil as much fresh sugar to blow as will cover them, and give them a thorough boiling; scum them, set them in the stove for twenty-four hours, and drain them; then lay them out to dry, after having dusted them very well

Note: In the scalding of green plumbs, you must always have a sieve in the bottom of your pan to put your plumbs in, that they may not touch the bottom; for those that do, will burst before the others are any thing warm

To put plumbs in jelly

Any of those sort of plumbs are very agreeable in jelly, and the same method will do for all as for one I could make some difference, which would only help to confound the practitioner, and swell this treatise in many places; but as I have promised, so I will endeavour to lay down the easiest method I can To avoid prolixity, and proceed as above, (*viz* plumbs in jelly) when your plumbs are preserved in their first sugar, and you have drained them in order to put them in a second, they are then fit to be put up in liquid, which must be thus. Drain the plumbs, and strain the sugar through a bag; make a jelly of some ripe plumbs and codlins together, by boiling them in just as much water as will cover them, press out the juice, and strain it, to every pound of juice boil one pound of sugar to blow very strong, and put in the juice, boil it a little, put in the syrup and plumbs, and give all a good boil; then let them settle a little, scum them and fill your glasses or pots

To make clear cakes of white pear plumbs

Take the cleareſt of your plumbs, put them into a gallypot, and boil them in a pot of boiling water, till they are enough, then let the clear part run from them, and to every pound of liquor, add as much ſugar, boiled to a candy height; then take it off, put the liquor to it, and ſtir all together till it be thoroughly hot, but not boiled, then put it in glaſſes, and dry them in a ſtove with a conſtant warm heat.

To preſerve green figs.

Take the ſmall green figs, ſlit them on the top, put them in water for ten days, and make your pickle as follows; put in as much ſalt into the water as will make it bear an egg; then let it ſettle, take the ſcum off, and put the clear brine to the figs, keep them in water for ten days, then put them into freſh water, boil them till a pin will eaſily paſs into them, then drain them and put them into other freſh water, ſhifting them every day for four days, then drain them, put them into clarified ſugar, give them a little warm, and let them ſtand till the next day, warm them again, and when they are become green give them a good boil; then boil ſome other ſugar to blow, put it to them, and give them another boil; the next day drain and dry them.

To preſerve ripe figs

Take the white figs when ripe, ſlit them in the tops, put them into a clarified ſugar, and give them a good boil, ſcum them and ſet them by, the next day boil ſome more ſugar till it blows, pour it upon them, and boil them again very well; ſcum them and ſet them in the ſtove, the day after drain and lay them out to dry, firſt duſting them very well

To candy figs

Take your figs when they are ripe, weigh them, and to every pound of figs add a pound of loaf ſugar,

wetted

wetted so as to make a syrup; put the figs in when the syrup is made, that is, melted, let it not be too hot when you put them in; boil them gently, till they are tender, and put them up in pots. To keep them too long candied they lose their beauty; but when you are desirous to use them, and you take any out of the pots, you must take care to add as much loaf sugar, boiled to a candy height, as will cover those remaining in the pots, but before you put the figs into the sugar, they must be washed in warm water, and dried with a clean cloth, let not your syrup be boiled above a syrup candy height. let the figs lie a day or two, then take them up, and lay them upon glasses to dry; they will candy in one hour's lying in the syrup, but it is better that they lie longer

To preserve green grapes

Take the largest and best grapes before they are thorough ripe; stone them, scald them, and let them lie two days in the water they are scalded in; then drain them, and put them into a thin syrup, and give them a heat over a slow fire; the next day turn the grapes in the pan, and heat them again the day after, then drain them, put them into a clarified sugar, give them a good boil, scum them, and set them by, the following day, boil more sugar to blow, put it to the grapes, give all a good boil, scum them, and set them in a warm stove all night; the day after drain the grapes and lay them out to dry, first dusting them very well

To preserve bell grapes in jelly.

Take the long, large bell, or rouson grapes, pick the stalks off, stone them, and put them into boiling water; give them a thorough scald, take them from the fire and cover them down close, so that no steam can come out; then set them upon a very gentle fire, so as not to boil, for two or three hours, take them out, put them into a clarified sugar boiled till it blows very strong, as much as will a little more than cover them,

them, and give all a good boil, scum them, boil a little more sugar to blow very strong, take as much plumb jelly as sugar, and give all a boil; then add the grapes to it, give them a boil together, scum them well, and put them up into your pots or glasses.

To preserve grapes in clusters, with one leaf, when you gather them.

Take the great Gascoyne grapes when they are green, before they be too ripe, and prick every one of them; to every pound of grapes add a pound and a quarter of sugar; make a syrup with the verjuice of the grapes strained; when your sugar is made clear and perfect, put in your grapes strained into juice, put them in a deep bason, cover them close, and set them on a pot of scalding water to boil; when your grapes are tender, take them up, boil the syrup a little more, and, betwixt hot and cold, put them in broad glasses or gally-pots, (which is better than glasses, as you must lay one cluster over another) then put a paper over them and tie them up.

To preserve mulberries dry.

Let the mulberries not be two ripe, but rather a reddish green, and tart, having prepared a quantity of sugar equal to the mulberries, and brought it to its blown quality, throw in the mulberries, and give them a covered boiling; the sugar also may be melted with the juice of mulberries to clarify it; when they have boiled, take the pan from the fire, scum it, and set it in the stove till next day; then take them out, drain them from the syrup, and put them up in boxes for use.

To preserve walnuts white

Take the largest French walnuts, when full grown, but before they are hard, pare off the green shell to the white, put them into fair water, and boil them till very tender; drain them and put them into clarified sugar, giving them a gentle heat, the next day boil some more sugar to blow, put it to them and give them a boil; the next day boil some more sugar to blow very strong, put it to the walnuts, give them a boil, scum them and put them by, then drain them and put them on plates; dust them and put them into a warm stove to dry.

Mrs Johnson's way of preserving walnuts black

Take the smaller sorts of walnuts when full grown, and not shelled; boil them in water till very tender, but not to break, so they will become black, drain them and stick a clove in every one, put them into your preserving-pan, and if you have any peach syrup, or that of the white walnuts, it will be as well or better than sugar; put as much syrup as will cover the walnuts, boil them very well, scum them, and set them by; the next day boil the syrup till it becomes smooth, put in the walnuts, and give them another boil, the day after drain them, and boil the syrup till it becomes smooth, adding more syrup, if occasion; give all a boil, scum them, and put them into the pot for use

Note They answer much better boiled up with the coarsest Lisbon sugar.

These walnuts are never offered as a sweetmeat, being of no use but to purge gently the body and keep it open.

To preserve garlick

Take a head of garlick, peel the cloves, throw them into spring water, give them just a boil, and preserve them as you do your apricots

Note. These are more proper for a cough

To preserve cucumbers.

Take little gerkins, put them in a large deep jug, cover them close down with vine leaves, fill the jug with water, cover it with a plate, set it in the chimney corner, a little distance from the fire, yet so as to keep warm, let them stand so a fortnight, then throw them

them into a sieve to drain; they will look very yellow, and will stink; throw them into spring water once or twice, to clear them, put them into a large deep stew-pan, or preserving-pan, cover them all over with vine leaves, put in as much clear spring water as will cover them; set them over a charcoal fire, look often at them, and when they are turned a fine green, drain off that water and put them into a fresh cold water; have your syrup made ready thus; to every pound of sugar, add one pint of water, the clear peel of a lemon cut in long shreds, an ounce of ginger boiled in water for a quarter of an hour, put the ginger and lemon peel to the sugar and water, boil it to a syrup, throw in your cucumbers, and give them a boil, pour them into the pan you intend to keep them in, let them stand till next day, and boil them again three times; when cold, cover them up, and they make as fine a sweet as is tasted

At the same time take large green cucumbers, full ripe, and cut them in four, long ways, put them into cold water, cover them with green vine leaves, and set them over a charcoal fire till they boil, take them off, throw them into a cold water, and repeat it several times, till they are a fine green and tender; then preserve them as above, or dry them as you do your other candied sweetmeats; either way they answer in tarts, mince-pies, or cakes, as well as citron

To preserve green almonds.

Take the almonds when they are well grown, and make a lye with wood, charcoal and water, boil the lye till it feels very smooth, strain it through a sieve, and let it settle till clear, then pour off the clear into another pan, and set it on the fire in order to blanch off the down that is on the almonds, which you must do in this manner, *viz* when the lye is scalding hot, throw in two or three almonds, and try, when they have been in some time, if they will blanch, if they will, put in the rest, and the moment you find their skins will come off, remove them from the fire, put them into cold water, and blanch them, one by one, rubbing them with salt, then wash them in several waters, in order to clean them; in short, till you see no soil in the water, when this is done, throw them into boiling water, and let them boil till so tender, as a pin may easily pass through them, drain and put them into clarified sugar without water, they being green enough do not require a thin sugar to bring them to a colour, but, on the contrary, if too much heated, they will become too dark a green; the next day boil the syrup and put it on them, the day after boil it till it be very smooth, the day following give all a boil together, scum them and let them lie four or five days, then, if you will dry them or put them in jellies, you must follow the directions as for green apricots

Note If you will have a compote of either, it is but serving them to table when they are first entered, by boiling the sugar a little more.

To parch almonds.

Take a pound of sugar, make it into a syrup, boil it candy high, and put in three quarters of a pound of Jordan almonds blanched, keep them stirring all the while, till they are dry, then crisp them, put them in a box, and keep them dry

To make chocolate almonds.

Take a pround of chocolate, finely grated, and a pound and half of the best sugar, finely sifted; soak gum dragon in orange-flower water, and work them into what form you please; the paste must be stiff, dry them in a stove

You may write devices on paper, roll them up, and put them in the middle

To make little things of sugar, with devices in them

Take gum dragon steeped in rose water, have some double-refined sugar seered, and make it up into paste;
some

some of your pastes you may colour, with powders and juices, what colour you please, and make them up in what shapes you like; colours by themselves or with white, or white without the colours; in the middle of them have little pieces of paper, with some pretty smart sentences wrote on them; they will in company make much mirth.

To make white loaves.

Take double-refined sugar, a little musk, and ambergrease, wet them with the white of an egg, beaten to a froth to the thickness of a paste; when beaten and tempered well together with a wooden spoon, take as much as a filberd, made up round and cut round the middle like a loaf; put them in the oven upon papers, taking care the oven is not too hot, for they must be perfectly white, only a little coloured at the bottom of the sugar; the longer they are beaten with the back of the spoon the better

To make sugar of roses, and in all sorts of figures

Clip off the white from the red bud, and dry it in the sun, to one ounce of that, finely powdered, take one pound of loaf sugar; wet the sugar in rose water, (but, if in season, take the juice of roses) boil it to a candy height, put in your powder of roses, and the juice of a lemon; mince all well together, put it on a pie plate, and cut it into lozenges, or make it into any figure you fancy, as men, women, or birds, and if you want for ornaments in your desert, you may gild or colour them, as in the wormwood cakes.

To preserve almonds dry

To a pound of Jordan almonds, take half a pound of double-refined sugar; blanch one half of the almonds, and leave the other half unblanched, beat the white of an egg very well, pour it on your almonds, and wet them well with it; then boil your sugar again,

again, dip in your almonds, stir them altogether, that your sugar may hang well on them; then put them on plates, place them in the oven after the bread is drawn, let them stay in all night, and they will keep the year round.

To make almond cakes for figures.

Boil a pound of double-refined sugar to a thin candy, blanch, with orange-flower water, half a pound of Jordan almonds; add the juice of one lemon, and the peels of two, grated to the juice, first boil your sugar and almonds together, keeping it stirring till the sugar is boiled to a proper height, put in the lemon juice, stir it well together over a slow fire, taking care it does not boil after the juice is in; make this into cakes, or what form or shape you please, and either gilt or plain

To make march pans.

Blanch and beat a pound of almonds with rose or orange-flower water, and, when they are firmly beaten, put in half a pound of double-refined sugar beat and seered, work it to a paste, spread some on wafers, and dry it in the oven, when it is cold, have ready a white of an egg beaten, with rose water and double-refined sugar; let it be as thick as butter, and draw your march pan through it, and put it in the oven; it will ice in a little time, and keep for use

If you have a mind to have your march pan large, cut it, when it is rolled out, by a gutter plate, and edge it about like a tart; wafer the bottom, and ice as aforesaid when the ice is rising, you may colour, gild, or strew them with comfits, and form them in what shape you please

To dry cherries.

Stone your cherries, and weigh them to eight pounds, put two pounds of sugar, boil it till blows very strong, put the cherries to the sugar, and heat them by degrees till the sugar is melted, for when the cherries come in it will so cool the sugar that it will seem like glue, and should you put it in a quick fire at first it will endanger the burning, when you find the sugar is all melted, then boil it as quick as possible till the sugar flies all over them; scum and set them by in an earthen pan, for where the sugar is so thin it will be apt to canker in copper, brass, or silver; the next day drain them, and boil the sugar till it rises; put in your cherries, give them a boil, scum them and set them by till the the next day; then drain and lay them out on sieves, and dry them in a very hot stove.

To preserve cherries liquid

Take the best Morello cherries when ripe, either stone them or clip their stalks off, to every pound take a pound of sugar, boil it till it blows very strong, then put in the cherries, and by degrees bring them to boil as fast as you can, that the sugar may come all over them; scum them and set them by, and the next day boil some more sugar to the same degree, put some jelly of currants, drawn as hereafter directed, for example, if you boil one pound of sugar, take one pint of jelly of currants, put in the cherries and the syrup to the sugar, then add the jelly, and give all a boil together; scum them, and fill your glasses or pots, taking care, as they cool, to disperse them equally, or otherwise they will swim all to the top.

To draw jelly of currants

Wash well your currants, put them into a pan, and mash them, then put in a little water, boil them to a mummy, strew it on a sieve, and press out all the juice, of which you make your jelly

Note Where white currant jelly is prescribed, it is to be drawn after the same manner, observing to strain it first.

To make cherry paste.

Take two pounds of Morello cherries, stone them press out the juice, dry them in a pan, and mash them over a fire; then weigh them, and take their weight in sugar beaten very fine, heat them over a fire till the sugar is well mixed, then dress them on plates or glasses; dust them when cold, and put them into a stove to dry.

Mrs Smith's way of preserving cherries in jelly

Take green gooseberries, slice them on the side, that part of the liquor may run out, put them into pots, and put into the pots two or three spoonfuls of water, stop the pots very close, and put them in a skellet of water over the fire, till the gooseberries have made a liquor as clear as water; half a pound of gooseberries will make this liquor; take a pound of cherries stoned, one pound of double-refined sugar beaten small; strew some at the bottom of your silver bason, and then a layer of cherries, and cover them over with sugar; keep some to throw over them as they boil, put to the cherries five or six spoonfuls of gooseberry liquor, set them over the fire, and boil them very softly at first, till your sugar is melted, and afterwards as fast as you can, scum it very well and carefully, when your liquor is jelly'd, it will stick upon your spoon, and then put it up; they do best half a pound at a time.

To preserve cherries the French way.

Take Morello cherries, hang them by their stalks one by one, where the Sun may come to dry them, and no dust can get to them; this must be in autumn, cut the stalks as for preserving, place them one by one in your glasses, scrape so much sugar as will cover them, then fill them up with white wine, set them in a stove to swell, and then use them.

To preserve cherries a cheap way

Take six pounds of cherries, and stone them; put half a pound of the best powdered sugar, boil them in a little copper, or other vessel, as most convenient; when you think they are enough, lay them one by one on the back side of the sieve, set them to dry in an oven that hath baked things, and when dry, put them in a stove to keep them so.

If any liquor be left, do more cherries as above, they will keep well coloured all the year.

Mrs Smith's way to candy cherries.

Take cherries before they are ripe, stone them, and pour clarified sugar boiled upon them.

To candy apricots, pears, plumbs, &c.

Cut your fruit in half, put sugar upon them, bake them in a gentle oven close stopped up, let them stand half an hour, and lay them, one by one, on glass plates to dry.

To preserve gooseberries green.

Take the longest sort of gooseberries the latter end of May, or beginning of June, before the green colour has left them, set some water over the fire, and, when it is ready to boil, throw in the gooseberries; let them have a scald, then take them out, and carefully remove them into cold water; set them over a very slow fire to green, cover them close that none of the steam can get out, and when they have obtained their green colour, which will perhaps be four or five hours drain them gently into clarified sugar, and give them a heat, set them by till next day, and give them another heat; this you must repeat four or five times, in order to bring them to a very good green colour; thus you may serve them to table by way of compote; if you will preserve them to keep either dry or in jelly,

you

you must follow the directions as for green apricots before-mentioned

To preserve gooseberries white

Take the large Dutch gooseberries when full grown, but before they are quite ripe, pare them into fair water, stone them, put them into boiling water, and let them boil very tender, then put them into clarified sugar in an earthen pan, and put as many in one pan as will cover the bottom, and set them by till next day, then boil the syrup a little, and pour it on them, the day after boil it smooth, and pour it on them; the third day give them a gentle boil round, by setting the side of the pan over the fire, and turning it about as it boils, till they have had a boil all over, the day following make a jelly with codlins, and finish them as you do the others

To dry gooseberries.

To every pound of gooseberries, when stoned, put two pounds of sugar, but boil the sugar till it blows very strong, then strew in the gooseberries and give them a gentle boil, till the sugar comes all over them, let them settle a quarter of an hour, give them another good boil, scum them and set them by till the next day; then drain and lay them out on sieves to dry, dusting them very much, put them before a brisk fire in the stove, and when dry on one side, turn and dust them on the other; when quite dry, put them into your box

Gooseberry paste

Take the gooseberries when full grown, wash them and put them into your preserving-pan, with as much spring water as will cover them, boil them all to a mummy, and strew them on a hair sieve over an earthen pot or pan; then press out all the juice, to every pound of paste, take one pound two ounces of sugar, boil it till it cracks, take it from the fire, put in the
paste

paste, and mix it well over a slow fire till the sugar is incorporated with the paste, then scum it and fill your paste-pots, give them another scum, and when cold, put them into the stove, when crusted on the top, turn them and set them in the stove again; when a little dry, cut them in long pieces, set them to be quite dry, and, when so crusted that they will bear touching, turn them on sieves, dry the other side, and then put them into your box

Note. You may make them red or green, by putting the colour when the sugar and paste is well mixed giving it a warm altogether

Gooseberry clear cakes

Gooseberry clear cakes are made after the same manner as the paste, with this difference only, that you strain the jelly through the bag before you weigh it for use

To dry currants in bunches.

Stone your currants and tie them up in bunches; to every pound of currants boil two pounds of sugar, till it blows very strong; dip in the currants, let them boil very fast till the sugar flies all over them, let them settle a quarter of an hour, and boil them again till the sugar rises almost to the top of the pan; let them settle scum them and set them by till next day, then drain them and lay them out, taking care to spread the sprigs that they may not dry clogged together, dust them very much and dry them in a hot stove

To preserve currants in jelly.

Stone your currants, clip off the black tops, and clip them from the stalks; to every pound boil two pounds of sugar, till it blows very strong, slip in the currants, give them a quick boil, take them from the fire and let them settle a little, then give them another boil, and put in a pint of currant jelly, drawn as directed before, till you see the jelly will flake from

the

the scummer; then remove it from the fire, let it settle a little, scum them and put them into your glasses, and as they cool take care to disperse them equally.

To ice currants.

Take fair currants in bunches, and have ready the white of an egg, well beaten to froth, dip them in, lay them abroad, sift double-refined sugar pretty thick over them, and let them dry in a stove or oven.

Currant paste

Wash well your currants, put them into your preserving-pan, bruise them, and with a little water boil them to a pulp, then press out the juice, and to every pound take twenty ounces of loaf sugar, boil it to crack, take it from the fire, and put in the paste; then heat it over the fire, take off the scum, put it into your paste-pots, or glasses, then dry and manage them as other pastes

To preserve barberries

Take a pound of barberries picked from the stalks, put them into two quart pans, set them in a brass pot full of hot water, to stew them; after this, strain them, add a pound of sugar, and a pint of rose water, boil them together a little, take half a pound of the best clusters of barberries you can get, dip them into the syrup while it is boiling, take out the barberries, and let the syrup boil till it is thick; when they are cold, put them into glasses or gallypots with the syrup

To dry barberries.

Stone the barberries, and use them in bunches; weigh them, and to every pound of berries clarify two pounds of sugar, make the syrup with half a pint of water to a pound of sugar, put your barberries into the
syrup

syrup when it is scalding hot, let them boil a little, and set them by with a paper close to them; the next day make them scalding hot, repeat this two days, but do not boil it after the first time, and when they are cold lay them on earthen plates, strew sugar well over them, the next day turn them on a sieve, and sift them again with sugar; turn them daily till they are dry taking care your stove is not too hot

To preserve or dry samphire.

Take it in bunches as it grows, put on the fire a large deep stew-pan filled with water; when it boils throw in a little salt, put in your samphire, and when you see it look of a fine beautiful green, take off the pan directly, and with a fork take up the samphire, lay it on sieves to drain, and when cold, either preserve it, or dry it as the barberries; if you frost them they will be very pretty

How to preserve rasberries liquid.

Take the largest and fairest rasberries you can get, and to every pound of rasberries take one pound and a half of sugar, clarify it, and boil it till it blows very strong, then put in the rasberries, let them boil as fast as possible, strewing a little fine beaten sugar on them as they boil; when they have had a good boil, that the sugar rises all over them, take them from the fire, let them settle a little, and give them another boil, to every pound of rasberries put half a pint of currant jelly, let them have a good boil, till you see the syrup hang in flakes from your scummer; then remove them from the fire, take off the scum, and put them into your glasses or pots

Note: Take care to remove what scum there may be on the top, when cold, make a little jelly of currants and fill up the glasses; cover them with paper, first wet in fair water and dried between two cloths, which paper you must put close to the jelly, then wipe clean your glasses, and cover the tops of them with other paper

Rasberry

Rasberry cakes.

Pick all the grubs and spotted rasberries away, then bruise the rest and put them on a hair sieve over an earthen pan, put on them a board and weight to press out all the water you can, then put the paste into your preserving-pan, and dry it over the fire, till you perceive no moisture left in it, stirring it all the time it is on the fire to keep it from burning, weigh it, and to every pound take one pound and two ounces of sugar, beat to a fine powder, and put it in by degrees, when all is in, put it on the fire and incorporate them well together, take them from the fire, scrape all to one side of the pan, let it cool a very little, then put it into your moulds; when quite cold, put them into your stove without dusting them, and dry it as all sorts of paste.

Note You must take particular care that your paste doth not boil after your sugar is in, for if it does it will grow greasy.

Rasberry clear cakes.

Take two quarts of ripe gooseberries, or white currants, and one quart of red rasberries, put them into a stone jug, and stop them close, put it into a pot of cold water, as much as will cover the neck of the jug, then boil them in that water till it comes to a paste, then turn them out in a hair sieve placed over a pan, press out all the jelly, and strain it through the jelly bag; take twenty ounces of double-refined sugar, and boil it till it will crack in the water, take it from the fire, put in your jelly, and stir it over a slow fire till all the sugar is melted; give it a good heat till all is incorporated, take it from the fire, scum it well, and fill your cake glasses, take off what scum is on them and put them into the stove to dry, observing the method directed before for clear cakes.

Note In filling out your clear cakes, and clear pastes, you must be as expeditious as possible, for if it cools it will be a jelly before you can get it into them

White rasberry clear cakes are made after the same manner, only mixing white rasberries with the gooseberries in the infusion

Rasberry clear cakes

Take two quarts of gooseberries, and two quarts of red rasberries, put them in a pan with about a pint and half of water, boil them over a quick fire to a mummy, throw them upon an earthen pan, press out all the juice, then take that juice and boil it in another quart of rasberries, then throw them on a sieve, and rub all through the sieve that you can; then put in the seeds, and weigh the paste; to every pound, take twenty ounces of fine loaf sugar boiled; when clarified till it cracks, remove it from the fire, put in your paste, mix it well, and set it over a slow fire, stirring it till all the sugar is melted, and you find it is become a jelly, take it from the fire, and fill your potts and glasses whilst very hot, scum them, and put them into the stove, observing when cold to dry them as pastes before

Rasberry biscuits

Press out the juice and dry the paste a little over the fire, then rub all the pulp through a sieve, and weigh them, to every pound take eighteen ounces of sugar sifted very fine, and the whites of four eggs; put all in the pan together, and with a whisk beat it till it is very stiff, so that you may lay it in pretty high drops, and when it is so beaten, drop it in what form you please on the back sides of cards, paper being too thin, if it be difficult to get them off, dust them a little with a very fine sugar, and put them into a very warm stove to dry, and when they are dry enough they will come easily from the cards; but whilst soft they will not stir; then take and turn them on a sieve, let them remain a day or two in the stove, then pack them up in your box, and they will,

44 THE COMPLEAT

will, in a dry place, keep all the year without forting them.

Rasberry jam.

Press out the water from the rasberries, and to every pound of rasberries take one pound of sugar; first dry the rasberries in a pan over the fire, but keep them stirring lest they burn, put in your sugar, incorporate them well together, and fill your glasses or pots, covering them with thin white paper close to the jam, whilst it is hot, and when cold tie them over with other paper

How to make a jam of cherries.

Take six pounds of cherries, stone them into four pounds of loaf sugar, and let them stand till the sugar is dissolved; then set them on the fire to boil very fast; when you find them stiff, shake in half a pound of sugar more, let it boil till it comes clear from the bottom of your preserving-pan, and then it is enough

How to keep fruit for tarts all the year

Take your fruit when it is fit to pot, and strew some sugar at the bottom of the pot, then fruit, and then sugar; so on till the pot is full; cover them with sugar, tie a bladder over the pot; then leather, and keep it in a dry place.

To keep grapes, gooseberries, apricots, peaches, nectarines, cherries, currants, and plumbs, the whole year

Take fine dry sand, that has little or no saltness in it, and make it as dry as possible with often turning it in the sun, gather your fruits when they are just ripening, or coming near ripe, and dip the ends of the stalks in melted pitch or bees wax; and having a large box with a close lid, dry your fruit a little in in the sun to take away the superfluous moisture, and lightly spread a layer of sand at the bottom of the box, and a layer of fruit on it, but not too near each other, then scatter sand very even about an inch thick over them, and so another layer till the box is full; then shut the lid down close, that the air may not penetrate; and whenever you take out any thing, be sure to mind the placing them even again, so you will have them fit for tarts, or other uses, till the next season; if they are a little wrinkled, wash them in warm water, and they will plump up again: you may use millet instead of sand, if you think it more convenient.

To keep cherries dry

Have ready a new stone jar, very clean and dry, with a mouth just wide enough to put your hand in; gather your fruit when full ripe and quite sound, and with great care lay your cherries in, with their stalks on, have a bung to stop it close, rozin the top all over, tie a string round it, and if you have a well, hang it so down as it may not come near the water, or touch the side of the well, and the well must be close covered; if you have not that conveniency, bury it at least three or four feet deep in the earth

To keep figs and stone fruit sound and fit for use all the year

Take a large earthen pot, put the fruit into it in layers, their own leaves being between them; then boil water and honey, scumming it till no more will rise, make it not too thick of the honey, and pour it warm on them; stop up the vessel close, and when you take them out for use, put them two hours in warm water, and they will have in a great measure their natural taste.

To keep strawberries, rasberries, currants, goosberries, mulberries, and damsons

Take new stone bottles, air them well in the sun or by the fire, to take away the superfluous moisture, and prevent its sweating; take off the stalks and put them into the empty bottles, by a fire, that may draw out as much of the air as may be, then suddenly cork them up, and tie down the corks with wire; let the corks be sound and not visibly porous, for if they be the air will come in abundantly and corrupt the fruit; then in a moderate cool place cover the bottles with sand, laying them sideways, and the closeness will preserve them

To keep grapes on the tree, or when pulled off the tree.

When they are come to their full growth, before they are quite ripe, make, for every bunch of grapes a bag of white paper, well oiled, close the top, that no rain can get into the bag, and they will keep good till after Christmas; or pull them when just ripe, and dip their stalks in melted pitch or wax, and hang them in strings across a room, so that they do not touch one another pears will keep the same way all the year.

To keep wallnuts, or filberds all the year.

Gather them when they are ripe, with the green husks on, bury them in dry sand, and mix the filberts with them

How to keep all sorts of flowers.

Gather them on a very fine clear day, at twelve o'clock, have ready a box and a little writing sand, place a layer of sand, then a layer of flowers, and so on, alternately, till the box is full; close the box that no air can get in

To green leaves.

Take little leaves of a pear-tree, keep them close stopped in a pale of verjuice and water, and give them a boil in some syrup of apricots; lay them between two glasses, to dry, smooth and cut them in shape of apricot leaves, for little apricot leaves are so tender that they will not endure greening; be sure they be got with stalks, and stick them in the apricots, close up the apricots as plump and natural as you can.

A grand trifle.

Take a very large china dish or glass, that is deep, first make some very fine rich calves-foot jelly, with which fill the dish about half the depth; when it begins to jelly, have ready some Naples biscuits, macaroons, and the little cakes called matrimony; take an equal quantity of these cakes, break them in pieces, and stick them in the jelly before it be stiff, all over very thick, pour over that a quart of very thick sweet cream, then lay all round, currant jelly, rasberry jam, and some calves-foot jelly, all cut in little pieces, with which garnish your dish thick all round, intermixing them, and on them lay macaroons, and the little cakes, being first dipped in sack

Then take two quarts of the thickest cream you can get, sweeten it with double-refined sugar, grate into it the rind of three fine large lemons, and whisk it up with a whisk; take off the froth as it rises, and lay it in your dish as high as you can possibly raise it, this is fit to go to the king's table, if well made, and very excellent when it comes to be all mixed together.

Calves-foot jelly for the above dish

Take four calves-feet, set them on the fire in a saucepan, or pot, that holds two gallons of water, et them boil fast till they are boiled to pieces, or two parts wasted, or till this jelly, by taking a little out,

be

be as stiff as glue; then strain it through a sieve, when cold take off the fat at top, then take two quarts of this jelly, one quart of mountain wine, the juice of six very large lemons, half a pound of double-refined sugar; and the whites of six eggs, first beat to a froth, mix altogether, let it boil, then run it through a jelly bag into a bowl, on a good quantity of lemon peel; then throw what quantity you want into your dish. pour the rest into a dish, so that you may cut it out when cold to garnish your trifle with

The floating island.

Take a quart of very thick cream, sweeten it with fine sugar, grate in the peel of two lemons, and half a pint of sweet white wine; then whisk it well, till you have raised all the froth you can, pour a pint or quart of thick cream into a china dish, according to the depth of your dish; take two French rolls, slice them them thin, and lay them over the cream as light as you can; then a layer of fine clear calves-foot jelly, or hartshorn jelly, then roll them over the currant jelly, then put the French rolls, and whip up your cream, lay it on as high as you can, and what remains pour into the bottom of the dish, garnish the rim of your dish with different sorts of sweetmeats, jellies, and ratafia cakes; this looks very ornamental in the middle of the table.

Calves-foot jelly.

Take a set of calves-feet, take the long bone out, split the foot, and take out the fat, boil these in six quarts of water, with half a pound of hartshorn, till it be jelly, which you may know by cooling a little in a plate, then strain it off, and scum the fat off, beat the whites of twelve eggs, add as much sugar as will sweeten it, the juice of six lemons, some mace, a little orange-flower water, and a pint of white wine; stir this all together over a stove till it boils; it must not be too sweet, nor

nor too sharp, strain it through a jelly-bag, and let it run on lemon peels to give it a colour.

Hartshorn jelly

Take half a pound of hartshorn shavings, an ounce of ising-glass; cut the ising-glass to pieces, and put it and the shavings to five pints of spring water, boil it to less than a quart, over a gentle fire, strain it, and let it stand all night to settle; melt the jelly, squeeze in two large lemons and a half, the whites of seven eggs, half a pint of white mountain wine, and sweeten it to your taste with double-refined sugar; then put all these ingredients upon the fire, stir it pretty much till it boils, but boil it very little; stir it well together, scum it through a jelly-bag, but let it not run very fast, if it does, put it in again; put lemon peel into the glasses, this quantity will make a dozen and a half of glasses.

N.B. When they are made for the sick, only sweeten them, and tincture them with saffron.

Jelly of apples

Take the softer sort of pleasant tasted apples, slice them very thin, take out the cores and seed, boil a pound of them in a quart of water, till a fourth part be consumed, strain it well, and to every pint and half put three quarters of a pound of sugar, with a little mace or cinnamon, and boil it up to a thickness, adding a quarter of a pound of ising-glass; then strain it again, and put it up for use.

Currant Jelly

Snip off the currants, put them into a jug, set the jug in a kettle of water, let it boil an hour, then throw your currants and juice into a fine lawn sieve, press out all the juice, and to every pint of juice put a pound of double-refined sugar; put them in your preserving-pan, set it over a charcoal fire, and keep it stirring till

till it is a jelly, which you will know by taking a little out to cool, observe to take off the scum as it rises, and when it is jelly'd and very clear, pour it into glasses, when cold, cut round pieces of paper that will just cover the jelly, dip'd in brandy, put white paper over the glasses, twisted round the top, and prick the paper full of holes with a pin.

Black currant jelly

Make it the same as the red currant jelly, only with this difference, make it with the coarsest lump sugar.

Note This jelly is never used in a desert, but it is a very good thing for a sore throat.

Rasberry Jelly.

Make it the same way as the red currant jelly, only put one half currants and one half rasberries.

Everlasting syllabubs.

Take three pints of the thickest and sweetest cream you can get, a pint of rhennish, half a pint of sack, three lemons, near a pound of double-refined sugar, beat and sift the sugar and put it to your cream, grate off the yellow rind of three lemons, put that in, and squeeze the juice of three lemons into your wine, put that to your cream, beat all together with a whisk just half an hour, then take it up all together with a spoon, and fill your glasses.

A second sort of syllabubs

Take a quart of the thickest cream you can get, made it very sweet with double-refined sugar, fine beat, grate in the yellow rind of two large lemons, first fill your glasses one-third full of sack, or any white wine sweetened, a little juice of orange just to give it a pleasant tartness, then with a whisk beat it up very well to a froth, take the froth, and with a spoon a spoon put it in your glasses as high as you can fill them, so keep it whisking up as long as it will from, and put it in your glasses; if your cream is thin beat up the yolk of an egg

A mock syllabub

Take a pint of sack and a pint of red port, the juice of a large lemon and a Seville orange, grate in the yellow rind of one of the lemons, and a little nutmeg; make it pretty sweet with fine sugar, take two quarts of new milk from the cow, make it blood warm, put it in a jug with a spout, hold it high, and pour it in as if milked from the cow; when it has stood five minutes, have ready a pint of good warm cream, and pour that all over in the same manner, it will be best to eat directly, but very good two or three hours after

A whim-wham.

Take a pint of sack and half a pound of Naples biscuit, put them in a deep dish or bowl, and let them stand ten minutes; take a quart of cream, whisk it well, pour it over the wine and biscuit, and send it to table directly, it must be made just as you are going to use it

You must mind to put in as much biscuit as will soak up the wine, and no more.

Newcastle curd and cream

Take new milk, and put it in the bason you intend to go to table; let it stand till it turns to curds, which may be one or two days after, eat it with cream and sugar, and it is very fine If your milk is good it will be two days turning

Rennet curd and cream

Take new milk and sweeten it, grate in nutmeg, and the yellow rind of a lemon; put in rennet enough to turn it to curds, which, if covered, will be in about two hours, then, if there is a quart, pour over it half a pint of thick cream, and send it to table

To make snow cream

Take a large deep dish, strew the bottom with fine sugar beat to powder, then fill it with strawberries, take some sprigs of rosemary, stick a large one in the middle, and several round about, to resemble a tree, then take a quart of the thickest cream you can get, and the whites of eight or ten eggs, then whisk it up for half an hour, till you have made the froth very strong, let it stand ten minutes, and with a proper thing take off the froth, throw it over your tree, and cover your dish well with it; if you do it well, it makes a grand pile in a desert

Almond butter with milk

To a quarter of a pound of blanched almonds, very well beat, put some new milk and rose water; take a quart of thick cream, and the yolks of twelve eggs, beat very well with a little of the cream, put the rest of the cream to them, then a quarter of a pint of new milk to the almonds, and strain it into the cream so often, that there is no strength left; strain altogether into a skellet, set it over a charcoal fire, and stir it till it come to a tender curd, put it into a strainer, and hang it up till all the whey runs out, then take six ounces of fine sugar, well sifted, and a little rose water, and beat all into butter with a spoon

Almond-butter jelly

Take a pound of almonds blanched, and beat fine seven yolks of eggs, and strain out the almonds, then set a quart of cream, or more on the fire, and when it boils up put in a little lemon peel, and

and the juice of a lemon, put it in a cloth, let it hang a day or two, and put it into dishes

Orange-butter.

Take the juice of twelve oranges, the yolks of eighteen eggs, double-refined sugar, sufficient to sweeten it to your taste, but not very sweet; set it over a slow fire, stirring it all one way till it grows thick, then put in as much butter as the bigness of a walnut, and a little ambergrease, keep it smooth with stirring, when it is thick, put it into little China dishes, being dipt in water first, that it may turn out the easier.

Fairy butter.

Take the yolks of two hard eggs, beat them in a marble mortar with a large spoonful of orange-flower water and two spoonfuls of fine sugar beat to powder, beat all to a fine paste, add a like quantity of fresh butter just taken out of the churn, and force it through a fine strainer full of little holes into a plate.

To make lech.

Take a quart of cream, boil it, and in boiling put in some dissolved ising-glass, stir it till it is very thick, and take a handful of blanched almonds; beat them very fine, stir them into the cream, and put into a dish, when it is cold, slice them, and lay the slices on a silver or China dish

Junkets.

Take a quart of new milk and a pint of cream; put it warm together, with a spoonful of good renner, and cover it with a cloth wrung out of cold water; gather your curd, and put it in rushes till the whey is run out, and serve it either with or without cream

Lady Leicester's Spanish pap

Take a quart of cream, boil it with mace, then take half a pound of rice, sifted, and beat as fine as flower, boil it with the cream to the thickness of a jelly, sweeten it with sugar, and turn it into a shallow dish; when cold, slice it, and you may eat it like flummery, with cold cream.

Cream curd

Take a pint of cream, boil it with a little mace, cinnamon, and rose-water, to make it sweet, when it is as cold as new milk, put in about half a spoonful of good rennet, and when it curds, serve it up in a cream dish.

To make lemon cream

Squeeze nine lemons upon a pound and a half of double-refined sugar, fourteen or fifteen spoonfulls of fair water, and set it on the fire till the sugar is all melted, put in the white of nine eggs, strain it and set it on the fire again; stir it all the while, till you see it begin to thicken, then put in orange-flower water, about four or five spoonfuls, take it off the fire, and put it into your glasses; you must cut some lemon peel in small strings, and lay in the bottom, after being boiled tender, this must be done over a charcoal fire.

Orange cream.

Do the same as the lemon above.

A second sort of lemon cream

Take one pint of thick cream, set it on the fire, keep it stirring let it simmer, sweeten it very sweet with double-refined sugar, keep it stirring till it is pretty cool, then put in the juice of half a lemon, with the peel squeezed in to give it a fine bitter,

keep

keep it stirring till it is cold, then stir it up high to bring a froth in the dish, this should be made early in the morning against dinner

To make clear lemon cream.

Take a little hartshorn jelly, and put into it the peel of two lemons, taking care there is none of the white, set it over the fire, let it boil, then take the whites of six eggs, and beat them well; take the juice of four lemons, grate in the peel to the juice, let it soak a little while, and afterwards put the juice and eggs together; put in such a quantity of double-refined sugar as will sweeten it to your taste, let it boil very fast almost a quarter of an hour, then strain it through a jelly-bag, and as it runs through, put it in again, till it is quite clear, after which take the peels of the lemons boiled in it, and cut them into each glass, stir it till it is half cold, and put it into the glasses

To make yellow lemon cream

Grate off the peel of four lemons, squeeze the juice to it, and let it steep four or five hours, strain it, and put to it the whites of eight eggs, and the yolks of two well beaten and strained; add thereto a pound of double-refined sugar, a quarter of a pint of rose water, and a pint of spring water; stir all these well together, and set it on a quick fire, but let it not boil, and when it creams it is enough

To make Spanish cream

Take three spoonfuls of flour of rice seeted very fine, the yolks of three eggs, three spoonfuls of fair water, two spoonfuls of orange-flower water, and mix them well together, then put to it one pint of cream, set it on a good fire, keeping it stirring till it is of a proper thickness, and then pour it into your cups

To make loaf-sugar cream

Take a pint of jelly of hartſhorn, put in a little iſing-glaſs, make it thick with almonds or cream, which you pleaſe; ſweeten it very well, and put it into tin pots; let it ſtand till cold, and when you uſe it, dip the pan in warm water, and take it out whole.

Imperial cream.

Take a quart of water, ſix ounces of hartſhorn, put into a ſtone bottle, cloſe and tied down, fill not the bottle too full, and ſet it in a pot of boiling water, or in an oven to bake, let it ſtand three or four hours, ſtrain it through a jelly-bag, and let it cool, having ready ſix ounces of almonds beat very fine; put into, it juſt ſo much cream as jelly, mix them together, then ſtrain the almonds and cream, and ſet all together over the fire till it be ſcalding hot; ſtrain it into narrow-bottomed glaſſes, let them ſtand a whole day, and turn them out; ſtick them all over with blanched almonds, or pine-apple ſeeds laid in water a day before you peel them, and they will come out like a flower; then ſtick them on the cream

Almond cream.

Take almonds blanched in cold water, beat them fine with roſe water and amber-greaſe ſteeped in them, take the yolks of ſix eggs, beat your cream, being boiled with mace, put in your almonds, and when well mingled, put in your eggs, taking care that they only ſimmer; when it is thick take it off, your cream muſt be an ale pint, half a pound of almonds, and ſix whites of eggs; garniſh with gilded almonds and dried citron.

Another of the ſame

Boil a pint of cream, beat an handful of almonds very fine with roſe water; take the cream off the fire and put it to the almonds, ſtir them together and ſtrain it, and ſeaſon it with roſe water and ſugar, let it boil faſt till it is thick, and ſerve it up

Piſtachia

Pistachia cream.

Peel your pistachias, beat them very fine, boil them in cream, if it is not green enough add a little juice of spinnage, thicken it with eggs, sweeten it to your palate, pour it into basons, and set it by till it is quite co'd

Cold cream

Take a pint of sack or rhenish wine, and a good deal of fine sugar, beat fine a quart of good cream, and a lemon cut round, a little nutmeg and cinnamon, and a sprig of rosemary; pour them all together, let them stand a while, and beat them up with a rod till they rise, take it off with a spoon as it rises, and lay it in a pot or glass, and then serve it up.

Codlin Cream.

Take twenty fair codlins, core them, beat them in a mortar with a pint of cream, strain it into a dish, and put into it some brown bread crumbs, with a little sack, and dish it up; so you may order gooseberries

How to make rasberry cream.

Take the whites of seven eggs, and seven spoonfuls of rasberry mash, put them both in an earthen pan, and beat it well with a spoon till it comes to a cream, or you think it looks white enough, then fill your glasses, this quantity will make about a dozen

How to make chocolate cream.

Take a quart of cream, a pint of white wine, and a little juice of lemon; sweeten it very well, lay in a sprig of rosemary, grate some chocolate, and mix all together; stir them over the fire till it is thick, and pour it into your cups

Almond

Almond cream.

Blanch almonds, bruise them small in a mortar, and strain them through a strainer with fair water, strain them again with thick milk, and with a quarter of a pound of sugar; put them into a pot, add a little salt, and set it over the fire; stir it well that it burn not to the pot; when it is boiled take it from the fire, cast a ladle of fair water into it, cover it with a dish, and let it stand; afterwards take a clean cloth of an ell long, let it be held strait and cast the cream upon it with a ladle, draw from under the cloth the water from the cream, pin the four corners together, and hang it up again

Steeple cream

Take five ounces of hartshorn and two ounces of honey, put them into a stone bottle, and fill it up to the neck with fair water, put in a small quantity of gum arabic, and gum dragon, then tie up the bottle very close, set it into a pot of water with hay at the bottom, let it stand six hours, then take it out, let it stand an hour before you open it, then strain it and it will be a strong jelly, take a pound of blanched almonds, beat them fine, and mix them with a pint of thick cream; let it stand a little, strain it, mix it with a pound of jelly, and set it over the fire till it is scalding hot, sweeten it to your taste with double-refined sugar, take it off, put in a little amber, and pour it into small high gallypots, like a sugar loaf at top, when it is cold pour them out, and lay cold whipt cream about them in neaps, taking care it does not boil when the cream is in

Sweetmeat cream

Take some good cream, and slice some preserved peaches into it, apricots, or plumbs, sweeten the cream with fine sugar, or with the syrup the first was preserved in, mix all well together, and put it into your basons

Stone cream.

Take a pint and a half of thick cream, boil it in a blade of mace and a stick of cinnamon, with six spoonfuls of orange-flower water, sweeten it to your taste, and boil it till thick; pour it out, and keep it stirring till almost cold, then put in a small spoonful of rennet, and put it in your cups or glasses, make it three or four hours before you use it.

Clouted cream.

Take a great quantity of new milk from the cow, boil it in a kettle on a charcoal fire, stirring it, and when it is just ready to boil, take it off and stir it a little, then lade it into a milk-pan, and let it stand at last twenty-four hours; then divide the cream with a knife, as it stands upon the pan, and take it off with a skimmer, that the thin milk may run away, then lay it into dishes, one piece upon another, till your dish be as full as you please to have it, keep it twenty-four hours before you spread it

Blanched cream

Take a quart of the thickest cream you can get, sweeten it with fine sugar and orange-flower water; then boil it, and beat the whites of twenty eggs with a little cold cream, take out the treads, and when the cream is on the fire and boils, pour in your eggs, stirring it very well till it comes to a thick curd, then take it up, and pass it through a hair sieve, beat it well with a spoon till it is cold, and then put it in your dishes

Almond custard

Take half a pound of sweet Jordan almonds, and three bitter almonds; blanch and beat them very fine with orange-flower water, and the yolks of six eggs well beat and strained, with a quart of sweet cream,

mix

mix all together, and sweeten it to your palate, set it over a slow fire, and keep it stirring one way till it be thick, then pour it into your cups, and if you would have it richly perfumed put in a grain of ambergreafe.

Orange custard

Take the juice of ten oranges, strain and sweeten them to your taste, dissolve your sugar in the juice over the fire, when cold, take six and twenty yolks of eggs, beat them well, and mingle them with a quart of cream, put the juice of ten oranges more in, and strain all together, keeping them stirring all the time they are over the fire, one way, for fear of curdling; when it is of a good thickness pour it into your cups

Plain custard

Take a quart of cream or new milk, a stick of cinnamon, four laurel leaves, and some large mace, boil them all together, and take twelve eggs, beat them well together, sweeten them, and put them in your pan; bake them or boil them, keeping them stirring all one way, till they are of a proper thickness

You shou'd boil your spice and leaves first, and when the milk is cold, mix your eggs and boil it you may leave out the spice, and only use the laurel leaves, or, in the room of that, four or five bitter almonds.

A second sort

Take a quart of new milk, the yolks of six eggs, beat fine and strained, and half a small nutmeg grated sweeten all to your palate, and either bake or boil them

A third sort

Boil a quart of cream, then sweeten it with powder sugar, and beat up the yolks of eight eggs with two spoonfuls of orange-flower water, stir all together

CONFECTIONER. 61

...ether, strain it through a sieve, set them on the
... and keep them stirring all one way till they are of
...proper thickness; then pour them into your cups,
...put them soon after in a stew-pan, put in as much
...ter as will rise half up the cups, set the stew-pan
...a charcoal fire, and let it simmer so as to have
... of a proper thickness.

A cream posset.

Take twelve eggs, leave out two or three whites,
...e out all the treads, and beat them very well into
... bason you make your posset in; add half a pound
...sugar, a pint of sack, and a nutmeg grated; stir
...and set it on a chafing-dish of coals till it is more
...n blood warm, take a quart of sweet cream, when
...oils pour it into a bason, cover it with a warm plate
...a cloth, then set it on a chafing-dish of embers till
...e as thick as you would have it, and strew on some
...cinnamon.

Orange leaves.

Scrape your Seville oranges, and cut off a piece of
...top, take out all the meat, and as much of the
...te as you can without breaking; boil them in wa-
...till they are tender, shifting the water frequently
... placing hot water in its room; let them stand in
... syrup all night, take them out and fill them with
...ick custard before it is baked; put on the lids and
...e them, and when they are cold send them to the
...e

Almond flummery

Take three ounces of hartshorn, put it to boil in
... quarts of spring water, let it simmer over the
...fi or seven hours, till half the water is consumed;
...le put it in a jug, and set it in the oven with hou-
...d read, then strain it through a sieve, and beat
... a pound of almonds very fine, with a quantity of

orange-

orange-flower water, when they are beat, mix a little of your jelly with it, and some fine sugar, strain with the rest of the jelly, stirring it till it is a little more than blood warm; then pour it into your basons or cups, and when you use them stick in almonds or small

Ising-glass flummery.

Take six ounces of ising-glass, put it in a quart new milk, sweeten it, set it over the fire, and keep stirring one way all the time, till it is jelly'd, pour into your basons, and when cold turn it out, you may put in orange-flower water, just as you like it

Oatmeal flummery

Take oatmeal, steep it in pure clean water till turns sour, stir it every day, strain it, and then put in a kettle over the fire, keep stirring it with a wooden stick one way all the time, till it is as thick as a hasty pudding, then pour it into your basons, and when cold turn it out; you may eat it with milk, ale, or wine, sweetened.

Bloomage

Take clear hartshorn and calves-foot jelly, make pretty sweet, put in a little orange-flower water, a little rose water, a little white wine, and the juice of orange, put in as much of all the ingredients as make it palatable, blanch some sweet almonds, pound them in a mortar with the orange-flower or rose water, as much as will turn the bloomage white and strain it well, stir all together till you find it, which you will know by taking a little out in a spoon, pour it into what thing you please to shape it in, and when cold turn it out and stick it with almonds, if it sticks, dip your bason or glasses in hot water

To make cheesecakes

Take a gallon of new milk, set it as for a cheese, and gently whey it; then break it into a mortar, to it the yolks of six eggs, and four of the whites; sweeten it to your taste, put in a nutmeg, some rose water, and sack; mix these together, set over the fire a quart of cream, and make it into a hasty-pudding; mix all together very well, and fill your pattipans just as they are going into the oven, which must be ready immediately to receive them; when they rise well up, they are enough; make your paste; take about a pound of flour and strew three spoonfuls of loaf sugar into it, beat and sifted; rub in a pound of butter, one egg, and a spoonful of rose water, the rest cold fair water; make it into a paste, roll it very thin, put it into your pans, and fill them almost full.

Potatoe or lemon cheesecakes.

Take six ounces of potatoes, four ounces of lemon peel, four ounces of sugar, and four ounces of butter, boil the lemon peel till tender, pare and scrape the potatoes, boil them tender and bruise them; beat the lemon peel with the sugar, then beat them all together very well, and let it lie till cold, put crust in your pattipans and fill them a little more than half; bake them in a quick oven half an hour, and sift some double-refined sugar on them as they go in; this quantity will make a dozen small pattipans.

Mrs Harrison's cheese-cakes

For the paste use a quart of fine flour or more, a pound of butter rubbed into the flour, with a quarter of a pound of sugar beat fine, two spoonfuls of orange flower water, make it into paste and put it into pattipans for the curd, take the yolks of twelve eggs beat in a pint of very thick cream, when the cream boils up put in the eggs, then take it off and put it in a cloth over a colander, whey some new milk with rennet for the other curd, when you temper them both together, take a pound of currants, three quarters of a pound of butter, half a

pound

pound of sugar, a quarter of an ounce of nutmegs, four spoonfuls of rose water, and bake them quick

Lady Leicester's cream cheese

Take a gallon and a half of stroakings, and put to it one quart of boiling milk, and one handful of marigold flowers, boiled in water and strained, then put in the rennet as the cheese comes; whey it gently down and put it in your vat and make your cheese, then turn it into a dry cloth into the vat, and put it into the press, when there an hour, take it out and shift it into dry cloths, so do five or six times, about five o'clock take it out and salt it, and put it into a dry cloth twice a day for four or five days, then put it into nettles fresh twice a day and keep it there two or three weeks, then eat it, it is a very good cheese.

Cheese cakes

Take tender curds, two gallons of milk, a quart of cream, and force the curd through a canvas strainer, add to this half a pound of good butter, a pint of cream, the yolks of twelve eggs, and two whites, put nutmeg, rose water, and salt to your own taste, then mingle these well together, and add to this a pound of currants washed, plumped, and dried, mix them all together and put them into coffins, and bake them in an oven or hot stove.

Cheese cakes.

Take the curd of a gallon of milk, three quarters of a pound of fresh butter, two grated biscuits, two ounces of blanch'd almonds pounded, with a little sack and orange flower water, half a pound of currants and seven eggs, some spice and sugar, beat them up in a little cream, till they are very light, and then make your cheese cakes

Orange cheese cakes

Take half a pound of Jordan almonds, beat them very fine, and put to them a little sack or orange flower water, lest they turn to oil; the yolks of eight eggs, and three whites, three quarters of a pound of melted butter, and the rinds of two Seville oranges, grated and well beaten, mix these all together and sweeten it to your taste; the oven must be as quick as can be without burning them, and a very little time will bake them.

To make rice cheese cakes.

Take a pound of ground rice, and boil it in a gallon of milk, with a little whole cinnamon, till it be of a good thickness; then pour it into a pan, and put about three quarters of a pound of fresh butter in it, then let it stand covered till it is cold; then put in twelve eggs, and leave half the whites out, and a pound of currants, grate in a small nutmeg, and sweeten it to your own palate.

Fine puff paste

To every pound of flour put one pound of butter, and the yolk of an egg. First take a quarter of a pound of the butter, and rub it in finely with the flour, then make a hollow in the middle of your flour, and beat the yolk of your egg very fine, or it will spot the crust, then put in as much cold water as will make it into a light paste, work it up light and roll it out, then divide the rest of the butter into five parts, take one and stick it into little bits all over, then shake a little flour all over, and roll it up round, and cut off a piece at the end, and lay on the middle of the roll, and roll it out again; do this five times and it is the finest puff paste you can make, and it will, when baked, fleak finely.

Fine paste for tarts.

Take a pound of flour, a pound of loaf sugar beat fine, and a pound of butter, work it up all together, don't roll it, but beat it well with the rolling pin for half an hour, folding it up and beating it out again, then roll out little pieces, as you want for your tarts

Paste for pattipans.

Take a pound of fine flour, a spoonful of sugar, three quarters of a pound of good butter, rub it all into your flour, then take the yolks of two eggs, the white of one, as much water as will wet it, beat them and pour it into the flour, and work it all together, then roll it out thin, and it will rise in baking.

Paste for a Pasty

Lay down a peck of flour, work it up with six pound of butter and four eggs, and make it into a stiff paste with cold water

Paste for a standing crust

To a peck of flour put six pounds of butter lay your flour in a large dish, make a hollow in the middle, put your butter in a saucepan of water on the fire, and when the butter is all melted take it off and put it into the flour hot, and with a wooden spoon or stick work it all together, then with your hands work your paste quick, and pull it all into little pieces, till it is quite cold, then work it up into a stiff paste, and form it into what shape you will and build your walls for a standing pye It requires a good deal of strength to work this crust

To candy any sort of flowers

Pick your flowers from the white part, then boil as much double-refined sugar to candy high, as you think

think will receive the flowers you do; then put in the flowers and stir them about, till you perceive the sugar to candy about them, then take them off the fire and keep them stirring till they are cold in the pan you candied them in, then sift the loose sugar from them, and keep them in boxes dry, or you may candy your flowers whole, just as you think best

To candy orange flowers

Take half a pound of double refined sugar finely beaten, wet it with orange flower water, and boil it to candy high, then throw in a handful of orange flowers, keeping it stirring, but don't let it boil, and when the sugar candies about them, take it off the fire, drop it on a plate, and set it by till it is cold.

To preserve hops with gooseberries

Take the largest Dutch gooseberries, and cut them across at the head, and half way down, and pick out the seeds clean, but don't break the gooseberries; then take fine long thorns, scrape them, and stick on your gooseberries, put in the leaf of the one, to the cut part of the other, and so till your thorn is full, then put them in a new pipkin with a close cover and cover them with water, and let them stand scalding till they are green (before your water boils) and while they are greening make a syrup for them, and take whole green gooseberries and boil them in water till they all break, then strain the water through a sieve; to every pound of hops put a pound and a half of double refined sugar, put the sugar and hops into the liquor, and boil them uncovered, till they are clear and green, then take them up and lay them on pye plates. and boil your syrup longer, lay your hops in a very deep gallipot, and when the syrup is cold pour it on them, cover them with paper and keep them in a stove for some time, afterwards in a very dry place

To

To preserve gooseberries whole without stoning

Get the largest preserving gooseberries, pick off the black eye, but not the stalk, then scald them, take great care they don't break, then take them and throw them into cold water, and to every pound of gooseberries put a pound and a half of double refined sugar, first clarify your sugar, to every pound of sugar a pint of water; and when the syrup is cold, lay your gooseberries single into your preserving pan, and put the syrup to them, set them on a slow fire, and let them boil, but not too fast, lest they break; when you perceive the sugar has entered them, take them off, cover them with white paper, and set them by till next day; then take them out of the syrup, boil the syrup till it begins to be ropy, scum it, put it to them again, and set them on a gentle fire; let them preserve gently till you perceive the syrup will rope, then take them off, set them by till they are cold, and cover them with paper, boil some gooseberries in fair water, when the liquor is strong, strain it off, let it stand to settle, and to every pint of that liquor put a pound of double-refined sugar, and make a jelly of it, put the gooseberries in glasses, when cold pour the jelly over them, and the next day paper them, wet and half dry their inside paper, to lie down the closer, put on your upper paper, and set them in a stove.

If you have a mind to make a little tree of them according to art, they will be pretty in a desert.

How to make wafers

Take a pound of fine flour, and eight eggs, beat them well together, put in a penny loaf grated, one nutmeg, two glasses of sack, a spoonful of yeast, better than half a pound of melted butter, and as much milk as will make it thick batter, let it stand three or four hours to rise; they must be well beaten, and when you have rolled them out thin, put them into any shape, and bake them.

A second

CONFECTIONER. 69

A second sort.

Dry the flour very well, either in a silver bason or pewter, over a charcoal fire; stir it often that it may not burn, and when cold sift it through a hair sieve, then make a thin batter with cream, a little water, sack, cinnamon, and mace beaten and sifted, with double-refined sugar, mix and beat all well together, and when your irons are clean and very hot, rub them with a little butter and a clean rag; then put them on and turn the irons, first one way and then another, till you think they are brown, which will be in a small time, take them off the irons, and roll them about your finger or a stick, and keep them in a tin pot near the fire, you must make them over a quick charcoal fire, or else they will not come off the irons whole.

To make sugar wafers.

Sift some fine sugar, put about two spoonfuls at a time in a small silver porringer or silver ladle, wet it with juice of lemon till it be a little thin, put in two drops of sack, with what perfume you like, throw it over a very slow fire, when a thin white skin rises, then stir it, and drop it on square papers as broad as your hands; if you make coloured ones, mix the colours as you do lemons, and make them as thin as you can, which you must do by turning your papers up and down, make it run, and spread it with your fingers; about two spoonfuls will make three or four wafers, they do best upon thin papers, that you may turn them round, and work them together as is used to be done for sugar; place and pin them up at one corner, in a warm place, till they are dry.

It must not be in too hot a place when it comes off.

To make comfits of various colours.

If you would have the comfits red, infuse some red saunders into the water, till it is of as deep a colour as you desire it, or if you please, you may use cochineal or syrup of mulberries

If

THE COMPLEAT

If green, boil some juice of spinage with the sugar;

If yellow, put saffron to the water you mix your sugar with

Note. They must all be boiled to a candy height, and then dried in your stove.

To make bean or almond bread

Take a pound of pure white almonds, and blanch them in cold water, taking care you part not the almonds; then take a pound of double-refined sugar, beat and sifted, then do your almonds, and slice them the round way, as you cut them strew on sugar, stirring them all together that they do not stick; be sure you have sugar to the last, and always stir them, for if they cleave to each other they will not be good, they must be put in an earthen bason, put in a small spoonful of carraway seeds, mingle well these together, and add a little gum-dragon dissolved in rose water and strained, put in also three grains of musk and ambergrease, dissolved in fine sugar, and the froth of two eggs beaten with rose water, make your froth as light as you can, and put in two spoonfuls of rice flour; when these are well mixed, lay them on wafers as broad as macaroons, and the thickness of two flat almonds open them with a knife or bodkin, let two or three pieces stick together, lay them as hollow and low as you can to make them appear in the best manner, and the quicker you lay them out the more hollow they will be, put them in a well heated oven, minding they scorch not, which will destroy their beauty; when they are half baked take them out, wash them with the white of an egg, scrape a little sugar over them, and let the egg be beaten to a froth, but let not your sugar be too gross, after set them into the oven about half an hour, then you may take them out, and when cold put them up

Note. We used to lay out bean bread upon whole sheets of wafers, and so cut round to the size; the quantity I used to make, was, one pound of sugar, one pound of almonds, six sheets of wafers, and one pennyworth of gum-dragon

You may leave out either the musk or ambergrease, if you please

How to make jumbles of almonds.

Take three ounces of almonds, blanch and cover them over with a cloth from the air, beat them in a stone mortar very fine, and, as you beat them, drop in a little gum-dragon laid in sack, to keep them from oiling; when they are almost beaten enough, take the white of an egg beaten to froth, one pound of double-refined sugar finely beaten, and put it in by degrees, working it with your hands till it is all in a paste; roll it out and bake it upon buttered plates, and set them in an hot oven.

How to make jumbles.

Take a pound of fine flour and half a pound of sugar beaten and feered, rub it in a piece of butter the bigness of an egg, a little mace finely shred, the yolks of four eggs, and the whites of three of them; beat them with rose water and a few carraway seeds, make it up in paste, with cream, in what shape you please, and bake them One pound of sugar and ten eggs make them extremely rich.

Lady Leicester's hollow gumballs

Take the whites of three eggs, squeeze in the juice of a lemon, and the peel grated in; with a whisk beat it up to a froth, have ready half a pound of double-refined sugar finely sifted, take off the froth as it rises, and put it into the sugar till it be wet and thick like paste roll it into what form you please, lay them upon paper, and put them in a moderately hot oven.

To make apricot jumbles.

Take apricots, pare and slice them into a clean dish, set them on the fire, and with a wooden spoon bruise them

them so that the pulp may be small, dry them on the coals, keeping them stirring till they are both dry and tough; lay them out in glasses in a stove, for two or three days, so cut them out in long pieces and roll them into rounds and shapes like tumbles, they must be rolled in double-refined sugar, and then dry them well in a stove.

To make orange jumble.

Take four oranges, let the peels be large, with thick rinds, take out all the meat, and boil them in three several waters till they are tender, and the bitterness out of them, then squeeze them hard, dry them in a coarse cloth, beat them in a stone mortar till they are come to a pulp, then take as much double-refined sugar, seered, as will work it into paste, and roll it into what shape you think proper

To make sugar of rasberries

Take what quantity of fine sugar you please, well beaten and seered; put it into a bason, set it over hot coals, and have the juice of rasberries infused in a pot of water, as you do your common cakes, then throw a little sugar among the juice, but not too much, that it may not dissolve the sugar but dry with it presently, let it dry as to a candy height, and it will keep all the year.

To make sugar cakes.

Take three pounds of fine flour, dried well and sifted, and add two pounds of loaf sugar beaten and sifted, put in the yolks of four eggs, a little mace, a quarter of a pint of rose water, and, if you please, you may dissolve musk or ambergrease in your sugar, mix all together, make it up to roll out, then bake them in a quick oven, and sift some sugar on them

To make sugar puffs.

Take the whites of ten eggs and beat them till they rise to a high froth, put it in a stone mortar, or wood en bowl, and add as much double-refined sugar as will make it thick; put in some ambergrease to give it a taste, and rub it round the mortar for half an hour; put in a few carraway seeds, take a sheet of weafers and lay it on as broad as sixpence and as high as you can, put them in a moderate hot oven half a quarter of an hour, and they will look as white as snow.

To make seed puffs.

Take gum-dragon and steep it in rose water; then take some double-refined sugar, seer and wet it with some gum as stiff as paste; work it with a spoon till it becomes white, roll it out upon white paper very thin, and cut it out in shapes with a jigging-iron, and bake it in an oven, taking care not to scorch it.

How to make little candied cakes

Take double-refined sugar finely seered, about a silver ladleful; wet it no more than will make it boil to a candy height, and put in what flowers you please, strew some sugar upon them, glass-drop them upon white paper, and take them off hot to avoid their sticking.

How to make tumblets.

Take of fine sugar and flour one pound each, eight eggs, with their whites taken out, and beat the yolks with two spoonfuls of rose water, take the quantity of a walnut of butter, which, along with the egg, put to half the quantity of sugar and flour, and mingle in the other half gradually. Some make tumblets thus take a pound of sugar, and mix with it the white of an egg well beaten, put to it a little grated lemon peel, making it in little balls, put them upon round papers, and do them in a pan over the fire till they are enough.

Ratafia biscuits.

Take four ounces of bitter almonds, blanch and beat them as fine as you can; in beating them, put in the whites of four eggs, one at a time, and mix it up with sifted sugar to a light paste; roll the cakes, and lay them on wafer-paper, or on tin plates; make the paste so light as to take it up with a spoon, then bake them in a quick oven

How to make sugar biscuits a cheap way

Take one pound of fine flour, one pound of powder sugar, a few almonds blanched and pounded, mix these with six spoonfuls of rose water, and the yolks and whites of eight eggs that are beat a full hour; when well mixed, put it into small tin pans of various fashions, and bake them only with the heat of the oven after the batch is drawn, and stop the oven very close

How to make Savoy biscuits

Take eight eggs, separate the whites from the yolks, and beat your whites till they are very high, then put your yolks in with a pound of sugar, beat this for a quarter of an hour, and when your oven is ready, put in one pound of fine flour, and stir it till it is well mixed, lay your biscuits upon the paper and ice them only taking care your oven is hot enough to bake them speedily

Savoy biscuits, a second sort.

Take twelve eggs, leave out half the whites, beat them up with a small whisk, put in two or three spoonfuls of rose or orange-flower water, and, as you beat it up strew in a pound of double-refined sugar well beat and finely sifted, when the eggs and sugar are as thick and white as cream, take a pound and two ounces of the finest flour that is dried, and mix with it; then lay it in long cakes, and bake them in a cool oven.

Lemon biscuit

Take the whites of four eggs, the yolks of ten, and beat them a quarter of an hour with four spoonfuls of
orange-

orange-flower water, add to it one pound of loaf sugar beaten and sifted; then beat them an hour longer, stir in half a pound of dry flour, and the peel of a lemon grated off, butter the pan, seer some sugar over them as you put them into the oven, and, when they are risen in the oven, take them out and lay them on a clean cloth; when the oven is cool put them in again on sieves, and let them stand till they are dry and snap in breaking.

Macaroons.

Take a pound of almonds, scald and blanch them, and throw them into cold water; dry them in a cloth, pound them in a mortar, and moisten them with orange-flower water, or the white of an egg, lest they turn to oil, afterwards take an equal quantity of white powder sugar, the whites of four eggs, and a little milk, beat it all well together, shape them round upon paper with a spoon, and bake them in a gentle oven on tin plates.

A second sort of macaroons.

Take a quarter of a pound of almonds blanched, and three ounces of sugar seered, beat these together with a little of the white of an egg and rose water, till it is thicker than batter; then drop it on wafer-paper and bake them.

Hard biscuit.

Take half a peck of fine flour, one ounce of caraway seeds, the whites of two eggs, a quarter of a pint of ale yeast, and as much warm water as will make it into a stiff paste; make it into long rolls, bake them an hour, and the next day pare them round, then slice them into pieces about half an inch thick, dry them in the oven, draw and turn them and dry the other side, and they will keep the whole year.

To make seed biscuit, the French way.

Take the whites of eight eggs, and the yolks of six eggs, put to them one pound of loaf sugar beat and seered, and beat them two hours; have ready fourteen ounces of fine flour double beat, sifted, and well dried in an oven, or over coals; when your oven is swept, and your plates buttered, put in your flour as fast as you can mingle them together, and lay them upon the plates, putting a little musk and ambergrease, finely beat into them; you must be very quick after your flour is in, and set them in a quick oven, this will make twenty large ones, laying out for each one spoonful

How to make Naples biscuits

Take a pound of fine sugar, and three quarters of the finest flour you can get; the sugar must be finely seered, and the flour three times, then add six eggs beat very well, and two or three grains of musk, with a spoonful of rose-water; heat your oven, and when it is almost hot make them, taking care they be not made up wet.

To make orange biscuit.

Take your oranges and water them two days, boil them tender, shift the water they are boiled in, and put them to another that is hot; when they are tender take them up, and put them in a cloth to dry, min*ing the meat be taken out of the oranges, then take their weight and half of double-refined sugar, finely beaten, let your oranges be beat in a stone mortar, strew your sugar on them as they are beating, and when the pulp is very small, and the sugar taken up with beating, then take it out, and lay it on glasses like your paste, minding to be quick in laying it out, for fear it grows rough and dries too fast, set them in an oven after manchets, and keep them in a stove to dry, beat the pulp of your oranges very

very small, or else they will look rough, dark, tough, and harsh

A rich great cake

Take a peck of flour well dried, an ounce of nutmeg, and as much cinnamon; beat the spice well, mix them with your flour, a pound and a half of sugar, some salt, thirteen pounds of currants well washed, picked, and dried, and three pounds of raisins stoned, and cut into small pieces; mix all these well together, make five pints of cream almost scalding hot, put into it four pounds of fresh butter, beat the yolks of twenty eggs, three pints of good ale yeast, a pint of sack, a quarter of a pint of orange-flower water, three grains of musk, and six grains of ambergrease, mix these together, and stir them into your cream and butter, then mix all in the cake, and set it for an hour before the fire, to rise, before you put it in your hoop, mix your sweetmeats in it, two pounds of citron, and one pound of candied orange and lemon peel, cut in small pieces; you must bake it in a deep hoop, butter the sides, put two papers at the bottom, flour it, and put in your cake, it must have a quick oven, and will take four hours to bake it, when it is drawn, ice it over the top and sides; take two pounds of double-refined sugar, beat and sifted, the whites of six eggs beat to a froth, with three or four spoonfuls of orange-flower water, and three grains of musk and ambergrease; beat these in a stone mortar with a wood pestle, till it be as white as snow, and, with a brush or bunch of feathers, spread it all over the cake, and put it into the oven to dry, taking care the oven does not discolour it; when it is cold paper it, and it will keep good five or six weeks

A plumb cake

Take two pounds ten ounces of the finest flour, well dried, two pounds of currants weighed after dried, picked, and washed; three nutmegs finely grated,

grated, three or four blades of large mace, ten cloves, a little cinnamon, dried and beat fine; mix all these into the flour, with two ounces of fine sugar, break into the bason the yolks of twelve eggs, and the whites of six, beat into them a pint of very good yeast, not bitter left it spoil your cake, strain it through an hair sieve into the middle of the flour, set over the fire a pint of new cream, and when it is boiled take it off the fire, put in a pound of new butter cut in thin slices, and as much saffron as will colour the cream; when the butter is all melted, and the cream not very hot, then pour into the flour as much as will make it like a pudding, but not too thin; never offer to mould it, but lift it up with your fingers till your flour be wet all over, flour a cloth all over, and lay it before the fire for a quarter of an hour to rise; then put it into a frame well buttered, and, with a knife dipt in flour, cut a crease acrofs, and prick it through to the bottom with a bodkin, and set it over a quick fire; set it in a quick oven, bake it a full hour, and draw it gently out of the oven, for shaking any cake will make it heavy; you may, if you please, add six spoonfuls of sack, some ambergreafe, citron and lemon; ice it as soon as drawn, and set it in a proper place, if you follow these directions, it will eat as if a great quantity of almonds were in it; but I seldom put in any citron

The icing for the cake

Take a pound of the best refined sugar, sift it through a lawn sieve, take the whites of two eggs well beat, with four or five spoonfulls of orange-flower water; put your sugar into the eggs, and never leave beating them till they are as white as snow, cover your cake all over, and stick some thin slices of citron, if you put any in the cake.

This cake hath been made for the best people in England; for it is an admirable one if carefully made.

A second

A second sort

Take seven pounds of flour, two pounds and a half of butter, and mix it with the butter, seven pounds of currants, two large nutmegs, half an ounce of mace, and a quarter of an ounce of cloves, all finely beat and grated; one pound of sugar, and sixteen eggs, leaving out four whites, put in a full pint and a half of ale yeast, warm as much cream as you think will wet it, and put sack to your cream to make it as thick as batter; beat also one pound of almonds with sack and orange-flower water, but do not let them be fine but grossly beat, put in a pound of candied orange, lemon, and citron peel, or more if you desire it very rich; mix all, put it into your hoop, with a paste under it to save the bottom. This was was given by one of the nicest housewives in England, and is as good as ever was made.

To make a very fine rich plumb cake.

Take four pounds of the finest flour well dried and sifted, six pounds of the best fresh butter, seven pounds of currants well washed, picked, and rubbed very clean and dry; two pounds of Jordan almonds, blanched, and beat in a marble mortar, with sack and orange-flower water, till they are very fine; take four pounds of eggs, leave out half the whites, and add three pounds of double-refined sugar, beat and sifted through a lawn sieve, with mace, cloves, and cinnamon, of each a quarter of an ounce; three large nutmegs beat fine, a little ginger, of sack and French brandy half a pint each, sweetmeats to your liking, lemon and citron; take a large broad pan, beat your butter to a cream before any of your ingredients go in, minding to beat it all one way, or it will turn to oil; put in your sugar, beat it well, and work in your almonds, let your eggs be well beat, put in, and beat all together till it looks white and thick, put in your brandy, sack, and spices, and

shake

shake your flour in by degrees, when your oven is ready, put in your currants and sweetmeats, and put it into your hoop; and it will take four hours baking in a quick oven.

Note As you mix it for the oven, you must be mindful to keep beating it all the time with your hand; and your currants, as soon as cleaned, must be put in a dish before the fire, that they may be warm when mixed. The above quantity bakes best in two hoops.

An ordinary plumb cake

Take three pounds of flour, a little ale yeast, a pint of milk, a pound of sugar, a pound of butter, and a little all-spice; make it into dough before you put in the plumbs, and work in as many as you please.

A pound seed-cake

Take a pound of flour, one pound of fine powder sugar, one pound of butter, eight yolks and four whites of eggs, as much carraway seeds as you like, first beat up the butter to a cream with your hands, minding to beat it one way lest it oil, then by degrees beat in your eggs, sugar, and flour, till it goes into the oven, bake it in a quick oven, and it will take an hour and a quarter baking.

Another seed-cake

Take two pounds of flour, two pounds of fresh butter rubbed well in, ten yolks and five whites of eggs, three spoonfuls of cream, and four spoonfuls of ale yeast, mix altogether, put it before the fire to rise, then work in a pound of carraway comfits, and bake it in an hour and a quarter.

A rich seed-cake

Take five pounds of fine flour well dried, and four pounds of single-refined sugar, beat and sifted, mix these

these together, and sift them through an hair sieve; then wash four pounds of butter in eight spoonfuls of rose or orange-flour water, and work the butter with your hands till it is like cream; beat twenty yolks and ten whites of eggs, and put them to six spoonfuls of sack; put in your flour, a little at a time, and stirring it with your hand all the time; you must not begin mixing it till the oven is almost hot, and after it is mixed, you let it stand some time before you put it into the hoop, when you are ready to put it into the oven, put to it eight ounces of candied orange peel sliced, with as much citron, and a pound and a half of carraway confits, mix them well and put it into the hoop; it must be a quick oven, and two or three hours will be sufficient to bake the cake, after which you may ice it if you please.

Little currant and seed cakes

Take two pounds of fine flour, one pound and a half of butter, the yolks of five or six eggs, one pound and a half of sugar, six spoonfuls of rose-water, nine spoonfuls of sack, three spoonfuls of carraway seeds, two nutmegs, and one pound of currants; beat the butter with your hand till it is very thin, dry your flour well, put in your carraway seeds, and nutmegs finely grated, afterwards put them all into your batter, with your eggs, sack, and rose-water mingle them well together, put in your currants, let your oven be pretty hot, and as soon as they are coloured they will be enough

Liquorice cakes.

Take hysop and red-rose water, of each half a pint, half a pound of green liquorice, the out-side scraped off, and then beat with a pestle, put to it half a pound of anniseeds, and steep it all night in the water; boil it with a gentle fire till the taste is well out of the liquorice; strain it, put to it three pounds of liquorice powder, and set it on a gentle fire till it is come to the thickness of cream, take it off, and put to it half pound of white sugar-candy seered very fine; beat this together as you do biscuit, for at least three hours, and never suffer it to stand still, as you beat it you must strew in double-refined sugar finely seered, at least three pounds; half an hour before it is finished, put in half a spoonful of gum-dragon steeped in orange-flower water, when it is very white then it is beat enough, roll it up with white sugar, and if you will have it perfumed, you must put in a pastil or two

The nun's cake

Take four pounds of your finest flour, and mix with it three pounds of double-refined sugar, finely beat and sifted, dry them by the fire till you prepare your other materials, take four pounds of butter, beat it in your hands till it is very soft like cream, beat thirty-four eggs, leave out sixteen whites, and take out the treads from them all, beat the eggs and butter together, till it appears like butter, pour in four or five spoonfuls of rose or orange-flower water, and beat it again; then take your flour and sugar, with six ounces of carraway seeds, strew it in by degrees, beating it up all the while for two hours together; you may put in as much tincture of cinnamon or ambergrease, as you please, butter your hoop, and let it stand three hours in a moderate oven

Saffron cakes.

Take a quarter of a peck of fine flour, a pound and half of butter, three ounces of carraway seeds, and six eggs, beat well a quarter of an ounce of cloves and mace together very fine, a penny'orth of cinnamon beat, a pound of sugar, a pennyworth of rose water, a pennyworth of saffron, a pint and half of yeast, and a quart of milk; mix all together lightly with your hands thus, first boil the milk and butter, scum off the butter, and mix it with the flour and a little of the milk, stir the yeast into the rest, and strain it; mix it with your flour, put in your seed and spice, rose-water, tincture of saffron, sugar, and eggs, beat all up with your hands very lightly, and bake it in a hoop or pan, minding to butter the pan well; it will take an hour and a half in a quick oven, you may leave out the seed if you chuse it, and I think it the best

A rich yeast cake.

Take a quartern and half of fine flour, six pounds of currants, an ounce of cloves and mace, of cinnamon, two nutmegs, about a pound of honey, some candied lemon, orange, and citron cut in thin pieces, a pint of sweet wine, some orange-flower water, a pint of yeast, a quart of cream, two pounds of butter melted and put in the middle, strew some flour over it, let it stand half an hour to rise, knead it well together, let it stand some time before the fire, work it up well, put it in a hoop, and bake it two hours and a half in a gentle oven.

Little queen cakes.

Take two pounds of fine flour, a pound and a half of butter, the yolks of six eggs, one pound and a half of sugar, six spoonfuls of rose-water, nine spoonfuls of sack, two nutmegs, and two pounds of currants; beat your butter with your hand till it is very thin, dry your flour well, put in your sugar and nutmegs finely grated, and put them all into your batter, with your eggs, sack, and rose-water mingle them well together, put in your currants, let your oven be moderately hot, and they will be baked in a quarter of an hour; take care your currants be nicely washed and cleaned.

Almond

Almond cakes

Take a pound of double-refined sugar finely seered, a quarter of a pound of the best almonds laid in cold water all night and blanched; take the white of an egg, put to it a spoonful of rose water, and beat it to the whiteness of snow, letting it stand half an hour, beat your almonds, putting thereto a spoonful of rose-water, a little at once, and the same with the egg; when the almonds are well beat, put the sugar in by degrees, and minding you wet not the paste too much whilst you roll out the cakes you must continue beating till all be used, and when your cakes are made, lay them severally on papers, with some seered sugar over them, bake them in an oven, as hot as for your sugar cakes.

Portugal cakes

To a pound of fine flour well dried, add a pound of double-refined sugar finely seered, take a pound of new butter, wash it in rose-water, and roll it till it is very soft, throw in the sugar and flour by degrees, till half in, working it with your hands, put in the yolks of six eggs, beat the whites with two spoonfuls of sack, and work in the other half of the flour; when the oven is hot, put in a pound of currants ready washed and dried; your pans must be ready buttered, fill them half full and scrape some fine sugar over them, the oven must be moderately hot, and set up the stone, you may make them plain.

Carraway cakes

To a pound of flour add a pound of new butter without salt, eight spoonfuls of good yeast, four spoonfuls of rose-water, the yolks of three new-laid eggs, carraway seeds as many as you please, four ounces of sugar, and some ambergrease, knead all into a paste, make it up into what form you please,

CONFECTIONER 85

please, and when they come out of the oven strew on sugar.

Shrewsbury cakes

Take two pounds of flour, a pound of sugar finely sifted, and mix them together; take out a quarter of a pound to roll them in, then take four eggs well beat, four spoonfuls of cream, and two of of-water, beat them well together, mix them with the flour into a paste, roll them into thin cakes, and bake them in a quick oven

Banbury cakes.

Take half a peck of fine flour, three pounds of currants, a pound and a half of butter, a quarter of a pound of sugar, a quarter of an ounce of cloves and mace, three quarters of a pint of ale yeast, and a little rose-water; boil as much milk as will serve to knead it, and when it is almost cold, put in as much carraway seed as will thicken it; work it all together at the fire, pulling it to pieces two or three times before you make it up

Whetstone cakes.

Take half a pound of fine flour, and the same quantity of loaf sugar seered, a pound of carraway seed dried, the yolk of one egg, the whites of three a little rose-water, with ambergrease dissolved in mix all well together, and roll it out as thin as a wafer, cut them with a glass, lay them on floured paper, and then bake them in a very few oven.

Bean cakes

Take weight for weight of fine sugar, and blanched almonds, cut in long narrow slices; slice some preserved orange, lemon, and citron peel, then beat the white of a new-laid egg, with a little orange-flower water, to a high froth; put so much of the

froth

froth into sugar as will just wet it, and with the point of a knife hold up your almonds, piling it round as high as you can upon a wafer, let some ambergrease be in your sugar, and bake them after the manner of a manchet.

To make gum cakes

Take gum dragon, let it lie all night in rose-water till it is dissolved, have double-refined sugar beaten and seered, and mix your gum and sugar together; make it up into a paste, then roll some up plain, and some with herbs and flowers, all the paste must be kept separately, your herbs and flowers must be beat small before you can make them into paste, but you may use the juice of the flowers and herbs only. I use sweet marjoram, red-roses, marygolds, clove-jilly-flowers, and blue-bottle berries, all clipped from the white; when you have made all your colours ready, have to every one a little rolling-pin and a knife, or else the colour will mix; first lay a white and then a colour, then a white again, for two colours will not do well, so roll them up, and cut them the bigness of a sixpence, but in what fashion you please, minding that they are rolled very thin.

To make honeycomb cakes.

Take your sugar and boil it to a candy-height; then put in your flowers, which must be cut, have little papers with four corners ready, then drop some of your candy on the papers, take them off when ready, and if they are rightly done they will look full of holes like honeycombs.

How to make lemon cakes.

Take the best coloured lemons, scrape out the blacks, and grate off the peel clean, put the peel into a strainer, wet what sugar you think will serve, and boil it to a candy-height, then take it off, and put in your lemon peel, when it boils take it off, squeeze in a little lemon juice, and drop them on buttered plates or papers, you may put in musk or ambergrease if you please.

To make lemon, orange, and flower cakes.

Take sugar finely seered, and wet it with the juice of orange, or any flowers you fancy, there must be no more juice than will make your paste wet and thick; set it upon the fire, when it begins to boil, drop it in little cakes, and they will come off presently; scurvygrafs done thus, is good against the scurvy; if it boils, you will spoil it.

Violet cakes.

Beat your sugar wherein gum hath been steeped, put in the violets and the juice, and to work it well together with seered sugar, and dry them in a stove.

How to make wormwood cakes.

Take one pound of double-refined sugar sifted, mix it with three or four eggs well beat, and drop in as much chemical oil of wormwood as you please, drop them on papers, and you may have them of various colours, by pricking them with a pin and filling the small holes with such colours; you must keep your colours separate in small gallipots: for red, take a dram of cochineal, some cream of tartar, and as much alum; tie them up severally in little bits of fine cloth, and put them to steep in a glass of water two or three hours, when you want the colours, press the bags in the water, and mix some of it in a little white of egg and sugar; use saffron for the yellow, prepared as the red; for green, mix blue with the saffron; for blue, put powder-blue in water

How to make cakes of flowers.

Boil double-refined sugar to a candy-height and then strew in your flowers, and let them boil once up; then with your hand lightly strew in a little double-refined sugar sifted, and then, as quick as may be, put it into your little pans made of card, and pricked full of holes at the bottom, you must set the pans on a cushion, and when they are cold take them out

How to make a cake, and leave out either eggs, sugar, or butter

Make your cake as you do the pound cake, leave out either the sugar, eggs, or butter, but then you must add thick cream instead of the butter; any of the three left out, the cake will be good

Brown almond gingerbread

Take a quarter of a pound of blanched almonds, beat exceeding fine with water wherein gum-arabick was steeped, with a few drops of lemon juice, as much cinnamon beat, and some ginger finely grated and seered, as to make it brown, make it sweet, and smooth it well, roll it out, and cut it in square cakes rolled very thin; dry it in a stove, or before the fire

A second sort

Take three pounds of flour, a pound of sugar, a pound of butter rubbed in very fine, with two ounces of ginger, and a grated nutmeg, mix these with a pound of treacle and a quarter of a pint of cream warmed together; then make your bread stiff, roll them out, and make them in thin cakes, and bake them in a stove or oven

Gingerbread

Take a pound and a half of London treacle, two eggs beat, half a pound of brown sugar, one ounce of ginger beat and sifted, of cloves, mace, and nutmeg, altogether, half an ounce, of very fine coriander and caraway seeds, half an ounce each; two pounds of butter melted, and mixed together, add as much flour as will knead it into a very stiff paste, and roll it out; cut it into what form you please, bake it in a quick oven on tin plates, and a little time will be sufficient

A second sort.

Take three pounds of fine flour, the rind of a lemon dried and beat to powder, half a pound or more of sugar, and an ounce and a half of beat ginger, mix all these together, and make it stiff by adding and working in treacle; make it into what form you please, you may put candied orange peel and citron in it, and mind you butter the paper it is baked on, and that it be baked hard and firm.

How to make whigs.

Take a pound of butter cut in slices and put it into a pint of milk, set it on the fire till it is melted, and take a quarter of a peck of flour, with some cloves, mace and ginger, then beat four eggs, a quarter of a pint of good yeast, and three or four spoonfuls of sack; when the milk is as warm only as though just from the cow, mix altogether to a paste, and let it lie half an hour to rise, then put to it a pound of carraway comfits, mould them into whigs, and bake them on papers; the oven must be hot as for manchets, and they will be almost as long in the baking

Light

Light whigs

Take a pound and a half of flour, and mix it with a pint of milk made warm, cover it, and let it lie by the fire half an hour, then take half a pound of sugar, and half a pound of butter, and work them in the paste, and make it into whigs, with as little flour as possible; and if the oven is quick they will rise very much.

To make artificial fruit

First take care at a proper time of the year, to save the stalks of the fruit with the stones to them; then get some neat pretty tins made in the shape of the fruit you intend to make, leaving a hole at the top to put in the stone and stalk, and they must be so contrived as to open in the middle, to take out the fruit, there must be made also a frame of wood to fix them in; and in the making of the tins, care must be taken to make them extreamly smooth in the inside, lest by their roughness they mark the fruit, as also, that they are made of exact shape to what they represent; because, a defect in either will not only give deformity to the artificial fruit, but likewise rob the artist of the honour she would otherwise acquire, and for which the lady would undoubtedly stand admired.

Then take two cow heels and a calve's foot, boil them in a gallon of soft water, till all boil to a jelly, when you have a full quart of jelly, strain it through a sieve, put it in a saucepan, sweeten it, put in some lemon peel, with perfume, and colour it to the fruit you intend to imitate; stir altogether, give it a boil, and fill your tins, put in your stones and the stalks just as the fruit grows, when the jelly is quite cold, open your tins for the bloom, and carefully dust powder blue, an ingenious clever person may make great improvements on this artificial fruit, as it requires great nicety in the doing it, a little practice will perfect them in it

CONFECTIONER.

To make ice cream.

Take two pewter basons, one larger than the other; the inward one must have a close cover, into which you put your cream, and mix it with what you think proper, to give it a flavour and colour, as rasberries, &c. then sweeten it to your palate, cover it close, and set it in the larger bason, fill it with ice, and a large handful of salt under and over and round about; let it stand in the ice three quarters of an hour, uncover, and stir it and the cream well together, then cover it again, let it stand half an hour longer, and turn it into your plate; your basons should be three cornered, that four colours may lie in one plate, one colour should be yellow, another green, another red, and a fourth white; but that depends on fancy, and what you colour them with; as any sort of fruit, saffron, or cochineal; and for the green, there are several sorts of juice; all must be well flavoured with different sorts of fruit, the white wants nothing but orange-flower water and sugar, three basons are made at the pewterers for the use above.

Some make their ice cream in tin pans, and mix three pennyworth of salt petre and two pennyworth of roach alum, both beat fine, with the ice, as also three pennyworth of bay salt; lay it round the pan as above, cover it with a coarse cloth, and let it stand two hours.

To make chocolate puffs.

Take half a pound of chocolate grated, and a pound of double-refined sugar beat fine and sifted, then with the whites of two eggs make a paste, and have ready some more sugar to strew on the tins; turn the rough side upwards, and bake them in a slow oven; you may form the paste into any shape, and colour it with different colours.

THE COMPLEAT

To make a pepper cake

Take a quarter of an ounce of whole pepper and half a gill of sack, mix and boil them a quarter of an hour, then take the pepper out, put in as much double-refined sugar as will make it like a paste, then drop it in what shape you please, or on plates, and let it dry

Oil of oranges.

Take a pound of sweet almonds well peeled, the flowers of lemons and oranges as much as you please, which you must divide into three equal parts, after this you must put a third part of the flowers upon a white linen cloth in a sieve, strewing upon the said flowers half of the almonds, which you must strew with another third part of the flowers, and then the rest of your almonds, which you must cover with the rest of your flowers, so that the almonds must always be in the middle of the flowers in the sieve, leave them together for six days, renewing and changing them every day; then beat the almonds in a mortar, and press them in a white linen cloth until they issue out clear oil, then stop it up close in a vessel, and let it stand in the sun eight days

Oil of jessamin and violets

Take sweet almonds well peeled and beat, with as much jessamin as you please, lay them rank upon rank, and let them lie in a moist place for ten days or more, then take them away and press out the oil in a press, this oil serveth for divers things, and in the like manner you may make your oil of violets and other flowers

Oil of nutmegs

Take of the best nutmegs to the quantity of what oil you will have, cut them in small pieces, and put to them as much malmsey as will cover them; put them in a glass for two or three days, beat them at the fire, and sprinkle them with rose water; press them in a press and you will have an excellent oil, good for many things, you must keep it close stopt in a vessel.

Oil of Benjamin

Take six ounces of Benjamin well beat into powder, and dissolved a whole day in a pound of oil of Tartar and a pound of rose water; then you may distil it with a fine pipe through an alembick, and keep it as an excellent thing.

Oil of storax

In like manner is made oil of storax; take what quantity of storax liquid you please, put into rose water two or three days, then distil it as the Benjamin above-said; first there issues out oil somewhat foul, and then an excellent oil

Oil of myrrh

Take eggs hard roasted, cut them in the middle; take away the yolks and fill them up with myrrh beaten into powder; put them in some moist place where the myrrh may dissolve by little and little; this oil maketh the face and other parts of the body soft, and takes away all scars

Oil of bay salt

Put the bay salt in an iron pot, and set it over a charcoal fire till it is dissolved and done running; take it off, lay the salt on a marble, and it will run oil; take four or five drops of this, rub it over your hands, and it will take all freckles and roughness off the skin

Note. In making of any of these fine oils to perfume the water, you must drop your oil on sugar and then they will mix.

Fine

THE COMPLEAT

Fine sweet waters

Take four pounds of damask-rose water, of lavender water, and spike water, three ounces each, the water of blossoms of lemons or oranges, the water of the blossoms of a myrtle tree, blossoms of jessamin, and of marjoram, of each half a pound, add of storax calamita, and Benjamin, a drachm each, and of musk half a scruple; mingle them well together, and keep it in phials well stopt six days; then distil it in Balneo Mariæ, and keep the water in a glass vessel fifteen days in the sun, and then it will be fit for use.

Another

Take of fresh flowers of rosemary two pounds, damask-rose water two pounds, and a scruple of amber put these into a glass phial well stopt for ten days, being distilled in Balneo Mariæ, and let it be kept in a glass phial stopt very close

Another

Take four pounds of the aforesaid water, two pounds of damask-rose water, and half a scruple of amber; mix these together, and keep them close stopt in a phial and put it in the sun for a month, and it will be fit for use

Another.

Take four pounds of damask-rose water, with six ounces of lavender-water, three pounds of jessamine flowers, and half a scruple of fine musk, keep them ten days in a vessel close stopt, distil in it Balneo Mariæ, and it will be extreamly good

Another.

Take the peels of oranges and green citrons of each half an ounce, a scruple of cloves, and six ounces of the flowers of spike, mix them all together with six pounds of damask-rose water, let them stand in a vessel covered for the space of ten days, distil them in Balneo Mariæ, and they will be extraordinary good

Another.

Another.

Take two pounds of damask-rose leaves, half a bottle of good amber, and beat them together; set them upon hot embers two or three days, and steep them ten days in ten pounds of damask-rose water, then distil it, and let it stand in the sun fifteen days.

Orange water.

Take the parings of forty oranges of the best sort, steep them in a gallon of sack three days, and distil the sack and peels together in an alembick; if you would have it very strong distil it in an ordinary rose-water still, put it into bottles, and drop in a little white sugar-candy; divide the oranges and sack twice.

Clove water

You may perfume it with any of the above waters.

Perfumed water

Take three handfuls of the tops of young lavender, and as much of the flowers of woodbine, full ripe and plucked from the stalks; then take as much orice roots as two walnuts and an half, an orange peel dried, and as much calamus as one walnut, and beat them all together.

To make rose cake to burn for perfume

Take three ounces and a half of Benjamin, steep it three or four days in damask-rose water, then of leaves half a pound, and beat them as small as for conserve, and put the Benjamin into it, with half a quarter of an ounce of musk and as much civet; beat them all together and make them up in cakes; then put them between two rose leaves, lay them upon papers in a place where no fire is, and turn them often into dry papers; when you use them, lay one on a coal, minding it is not too hot.

To perfume roses.

Take damask-rose buds and cut off the whites, then take orange-flower or rose water, wherein Benjamin, storax, lignum rhodium, civet, and musk, have been steeped; dip some leaves therein, and stick a clove into every rose bud; dry them betwixt two papers, and they will fall asunder; this perfume will last seven years.

How to make fine sweet water.

Take sweet marjoram, lavender, rosemary muscovy, maudillon balon, fine walnut leaves, damask roses, and pinks, of all a like quantity, and enough to fill the still, then take of the best orange and damask-rose powder, and storax, of each two ounces, strew one handful or two of the powder upon your herbs, and distil them upon a soft fire; tie a little musk in a piece of lawn, and hang it in a glass your water drops into, when it is all distilled, take out the cakes, and mix them with the powders that are left, lay them among your cloaths, or with sweet oils, and burn them for perfumes.

Some perfume roses thus.

Take your rose leaves, cut them from the whites, and sprinkle them with the aforesaid water, putting some powder of cloves among them, and when dry, put them up in bags to sweeten your cloaths.

Another way.

Take your rose leaves, and as you pull them lay them so that they touch not one another, turning them every day; when they are very dry put them up in a wide mouthed glass, and tie them up close, these roses thus dried will keep their perfect colour.

How to make Hungary water.

Take rosemary flowers, and put a good quantity of them into a wide mouthed glass, then put to them no more

more spirit of sack than will be strong of your flowers, cork them close, and let them stand ten days at least, stirring it frequently; then distil it in an alembick, and keep it for use.

Lavender water.

Take a quart of spirits of wine and put in the essence.

How to make ratafia.

To every gallon of brandy put a quart of the best orange-flower water, and a quart of good French wine; you must also take care your brandy is extremely fine, and of a good age; put in four hundred apricot stones, and a pound and a quarter of white sugar-candy; just crack the stones, and put them in, with the shells, into a bottle, stop it very close, seal it down, and put it in the sun for six weeks, take it in every night, and in wet weather, and whenever you take it in, or set it out, shake it well about; after the time is expired, let it settle, and rack it off when it is perfectly fine.

Surfeit water.

Take a gallon of brandy, half a pound of white sugar-candy beat small, one pound and a half of raisins of the sun stoned, a quarter of a pound of dates shread, a quarter of a pound of whole mace, with an ounce of nutmeg sliced, half an ounce of anniseeds, carraway seeds, and coriander seeds; half an ounce of cardimum bruised, and as many poppies as will colour it well, these all mixed together, add a large sprig of angelica, rue, wormwood, spermint, balm, rosemary, marygolds, sage, clove-jilly flowers, burrage, cowslips, and rosemary flowers, of each a handful, let them stand nine days close stopped, then strain it thro' a fine bag, and bottle it up.

Note. To the ingredients above prescribed, put a gallon of brandy, and let it stand nine days, distil it in an alembick, and it will make an excellent water: Infuse these things in a wide mouthed glass

THE COMPLEAT

Plague water

Take rosa solis, agrimony, betony, scabius, centaury tops, scordium, balm, rue, wormwood, mugwort, celandine, rosemary, marygold leaves, brown sage, burnet, carduus, and dragons, of each a large handful; angelica roots, piony roots, tormentil roots, elecampane roots, and liquorice, of each one ounce, cut the herbs, slice the roots, and put them all into an earthen pot, add to them a gallon of white wine, and a quart of brandy, let them steep two days close covered, then distil it in an ordinary still over a gentle fire, and sweeten it as you think proper

Walnut water

Take a peck of walnuts in July and beat them pretty small, putting to them two quarts of clove-gilly flowers, two quarts of poppy flowers, two quarts of cowslip flowers dried, two quarts of marygold flowers, two quarts of sage flowers, and two quarts of burrage flowers; add to these, two ounces of mace well beat, two ounces of nutmegs bruised, and an ounce of cinnamon well beat; steep all these in a pot, with a gallon of brandy and two gallons of sack, let it stand twenty-four hours, and distil it off

Juniper berries

Take of the best juniper berries twelve ounces, proof spirits of wine three gallons, a sufficient quantity of water, and distil them. you may sweeten it with sugar. It is an excellent remedy against wind in the stomach and bowels, powerfully provokes urine, and is therefore a good diuretic in the gravel and the jaundice; you may distil it a second time, only by adding the same quantity of berries

Cardamum water

Take pimento, carraway and coriander seeds, and lemon peel, of each four ounces; proof spirits three gallons,

gallons, and a sufficient quantity of water; distil it, and sweeten it with one pound and a half of sugar; this is a cheap and good cordial, and may be used in all cases where a stomachic cordial is necessary.

Nutmeg water.

Take and bruise half a pound of nutmegs, an ounce of orange peel, spirits of wine rectified three gallons, and a sufficient quantity of water; distil and sweeten them with two pounds of loaf sugar. It is an excellent cephalic and stomachic cordial, it helps the memory and strengthens the eyesight.

Mint, balm, or pennyroyal water.

Take four pounds of dried mint, (three pounds of any of the other herbs are sufficient) two gallons and a half of proof spirits, and three gallons of water; distil them, and sweeten the water with one pound and a half of sugar.

Citron water.

Take eighteen ounces of the best lemon peel bruised, nine ounces of orange peel bruised, nutmegs bruised one quarter of a pound, and three gallons of proof spirits, macerate and distil them, sweeten the water with two pounds of double-refined sugar, and keep it for use.

A second sort.

Take the outward yellow rind of twelve lemons, and half an ounce of cardamum seeds a little bruised; let these steep three days in the best French brandy, close stopt, in the mean time take of double-refined sugar one pound and a half, and boil it with a pint and a half of spring water, boil it gently to a syrup, scum it, and when it is cold mix it with brandy, adding the juice of three lemons, let it run through a bag once or twice, till it is fine and clear, then put it into pint bottles.

Note. You must be mindful that the brandy is free from adulteration, and the lemons favour not the least of sweetness, or are any ways musty.

Cinnamon water

Take two pounds of cinnamon and bruise it, half a pound of citron and orange peel, a quarter of an ounce of coriander seed, steeped two days in three gallons of malaga sack; distil them in a worm still, and sweeten it with sugar dissolved in red-rose water; this water hath been highly esteemed for the taste.

Orange water.

To every two quarts of sack add twelve oranges, chop and steep them twelve hours, distil them in a glass still, sweeten it with very fine double-refined sugar dissolved in red-rose water; put one handful of angelica into the still with the oranges.

Milk water.

Take balm, mint, carduus, angelica, rue, wormwood, rosemary, of each half a pound, and sweeten them; distil them with two gallons of milk just taken from the cow, in an alembick, with an iron pot; put in with the herbs a quart of water, first heat it, then carefully pour in the milk all round on the herbs, by a pint at a time, till all be poured in; this must be done in an iron pot covered with the still head, and shut close, when it boils, lower the fire a little.

N B Do not put quite the quantity of mint and wormwood, but as much of the balm and sweet meadow as will make up the quantity.

Clary water.

Take a quart of burrage water, put it in an earthen jug, and fill it with two or three quarts of clary flowers, fresh gathered; let it infuse an hour over the fire in a kettle of water, then take out the flowers, and

and put in as many fresh flowers, and so do for six or seven times together, then add to that water, two quarts of the best sack, a gallon of fresh flowers, and two pounds of white sugar candy beat small, distil it off in a cold still, mix all the water together, and when it is distilled sweeten it to your taste with the finest sugar, this is a very wholsome water, and extreamly pleasant tasted if corked, well and kept close

Lady Hewet's water.

Take red sage, betony, spermint, unset hyssop, setwell, thyme, balm, pennyroyal, calendine, water-cresses, heart's ease, lavender, angelica, germander, calamita, tamarisk, coltsfoot, avens, valerian, saxi-frage, pimpernal, vervain, parsley, rosemary, savory, scabius, agrimony, mother thyme, wild marjoram, Roman wormwood, carduus benedictus, pelliiary of the wall, field-daisies, with their flowers and leaves, of each of these herbs a handful; after they are pickled and washed, add of rue, yellow comfry-plaintain, camomile, maiden hair, sweet marjoram, and dragons, a handful of each, before they are washed or picked, of red-rose leaves and cowslip flowers half a peck each, rosemary flowers a quarter of a peck; hartshorn two ounces, juniper berries one drachm, China roots one ounce, comfry roots sliced, anniseeds, fennel seeds, carraway seeds, nutmegs, ginger, cinnamon, pepper, spikenard, parsley seeds, cloves, and mace, aromaticum rosarum, three drachms, sassafras sliced half an ounce, elecampane roots, mellilot flowers, calamus aromaticus, cardamums, lignum aloes, rhubarb sliced, thin galingal, veronica, lodericum, cubeb grains, of each of these two drachms, the cordial bezoar thirty grains, musk twenty-four grains, amber-grease twenty grains, flour of coral 2 drachms, flour of amber one drachm, flour of pearl two drachms, four leaves of gold, two drachms of saffron in a little bag, and white sugar-candy one pound; wash the herbs and hang them in a cloth till dry; cut and put them into an earthen pot, and in the midst of the herbs put the seeds, spices and drugs, all being weel bruised, then put thereto such a quantity of sherry sack as will cover them, and let them steep twenty-four hours, then put it in an alembick, and make two distillings of it, and from each draw three pints of water, mix all together, and put it into quart bottles; then divide the cordials into three parts, and put into each bottle of water a like quantity. Shake it often together at the first, and the longer you keep it the better it will be. There never was a better cordial in cases of the greatest illness, two or three spoonfuls almost revive from death.

To make treacle water.

Take the juice of three walnuts, four pounds of rue, carduus, marygolds, and balm, of each three pounds; roots of butterbur half a pound, roots of burdock one pound, angelica and masterworth of each half a pound, leaves of scordium six handfuls, Venice treacle and mithridate of each half a pound, old Canary wine one pound, white-wine vinegar six pounds, juice of lemons six pounds, distil these in an alembick, and on any illness take four spoonfuls upon going to bed.

Palsey water.

Take of sage, rosemary, and betony flowers, each half a handful, burrage and buglois flowers, of each half a handful; lilies of the valley and cowslip flowers of each four or five handfuls, steep these in the best spirit of sack, and add some balm, spike flowers, mother wort, bay leaves, leaves of an orange tree, and their flowers, then put in citron peel, piony seeds, and cinnamon, of each half an ounce, nutmegs, cardamums, mace, cubebs, yellow sanders, of each half an ounce; lignum aloes one drachm; make all these into powder, and add half a pound of jujabes with the stones taken out; then add pearl prepared, Smaragde's musk, and saffron, of each ten grains; ambergrease

bergrease one scruple, red roses dried one ounce, and dry lavender flowers, stripped from their stalks, will fill a gallon glass; steep all these a month, and distil them in an alembick very carefully, after it is distilled, hang it in a bag with the following ingredients, pearl, Smaragde's musk, and saffron, of each ten grains, ambergrease one scruple, red roses dried, red and yellow sanders, of each one ounce, hang them in a white sarsnet bag in the water, close stopped.

Hysterical water.

Take zedoary, roots of lovage, seeds of wild parsnips, of each two ounces, roots of single piony four ounces, misletoe of the oak three ounces, myrrh a quarter of an ounce, and castor half an ounce; beat all these together, and add to them a quarter of a pound of dried millepedes, pour on them three quarts of mugwort water, and two quarts of brandy; let them stand in a close vessel eight days, and distil it in a cold still, draw off nine pints of water, sweeten it to your taste, and mix all together. This is an excellent water to prevent fits, or to be taken in faintings.

Black-cherry water for children.

Take six pounds of black cherries, and bruise them small, then put to them the tops of rosemary, sweet marjoram, spearmint, angelica, balm, and marygold flowers, of each a handful, dried violets one ounce, annifeeds, and sweet-fennel seeds, of each half an ounce bruised, cut the herbs small, and mix all together; distil them off in a cold still, and you will find it an excellent water for children, giving them two or three spoonfuls at a time.

F 4   *Lady*

THE COMPLEAT

Lady Allen's water.

Take of palm, rosemary, sage, carduus, wormwood, cragons, scordium, mugwort, scabius, tormentil roots and leaves, angelica roots and leaves, betony flowers and leaves, centaury tops, pimpernel, wood or other sorrel, rue, agrimony, and rosa solis, of every one of these half a pound, liquorice four ounces, and elecampane roots two ounces, wash the herbs, shake and dry them in a cloth, shred them, slice the roots, put all in three gallons of the best white wine, and let them stand close covered two days and nights, stirring them morning and evening, then take out some of the herbs, lightly squeezing them with your hands into the still, fill the still with the herbs and the wine, let them stand twelve hours in a cold still, and distil them through an alembick till the herbs and wine are out, mix the water of each still together, sweeten it, preserving some unsweetened as a preservative to women in their illness. This is a most excellent water.

How to make all sorts of herb waters

Gather your herbs of a very fine clear day, chop them well, and put them in an earthen pan, wash them with sack, or if you do not chuse that expence, wash them with water, let them stand twenty-four hours, distil them in a cold still over a gentle fire, and you may put a piece of white sugar-candy into the bottom for it to drop on

Orange-mint water

Take a still full of orange mint, distill it in a cold still, and in the water put fresh orange mint, distil it again, and put your bottles into the still unstopped a spoonful of this water put into a glass of spring water, will perfume it as excellently as the orange-flower water.

To make bitters.

Take a quarter of a hundred of Seville oranges, peel them, and put the clear peel to a gallon of brandy, a quarter of an ounce of saffron, one ounce of cochineal, half an ounce of gentian root, and half an ounce of snake root; let them lie in the brandy for a month, pour it clear off, and it will be fit for use

Cherry brandy

Take of black and morello cherries a like quantity, fill your jar or bottle full, to every dozen of cherries put in half a pound of either plumb or apricot kernels, fill it up with French brandy, and the longer it stands the better it will be

Currant brandy

Fill the bottle or pan with the fruit as above, then fill it up with brandy

Rasberry brandy

Do the same way as you do the currant brandy.

Sir John Cope's shrub

Take two gallons of brandy, two dozen of Genoa lemons, and peel the yellow rinds very thin; throw away all the whites of the rinds, slice the lemons, and throw away the stones, then let the yellow rind, and the lemons so sliced, infuse in the brandy five or six days, let them drain through a thick flannel, and put to the brandy a gallon of white wine or rhenish, with six pounds of white sugar; bottle it up, and let it be close sealed

Sir John Cope's cyder, good and fit for drinking in two or three days.

Take the usual quantity of apples, pound them, and pour three gallons of water on each bushel;

put them into a tub, or any other wood veſſel, with a ſpigot near the bottom; let them infuſe twenty-four hours, then, without preſſing or jogging the veſſel, draw off the liquor into bottles, which after two or three days will be clear and fit to drink, but it will be too briſk if kept much longer; I ſuppoſe it may be convenient to faſten a ſmall baſket ſuch as brewers uſe, to the end of the foſſet, to keep the apples from ſtopping it, this liquor is moſt properly called pumparkine, and not cyder, and has been tried with one buſhel of apples by Sir John Cope

Mr. Bentham's cyder.

Take your apples and beat them in a wooden trough, till they are well maſhed; then put them into a clean hair bag, and ſqueeze and preſs out the juice, and let it run into a clean veſſel, ſo put it up into a barrel you intend to keep it in it is beſt to be thick, I made three kilderkins and ten gallons of cyder with ten buſhels of pippins and fourteen buſhels of other apples; you muſt clay up your veſſel, as you do beer, the next morning

How to make perry

Take pears that have a vinous juice, ſuch as gooſeberry pears, horſe pears, both the red and white, the john and choke pears, and other pears of the like kind, take the reddeſt of the ſort, let them be ripe, but not too ripe, and grind them as you do apples for cyder; work it off in the ſame manner; if your pears are of a ſweet taſte mix a few crabs with them

Uſquebaugh

Take ten gallons of good malt ſpirits, anniſeeds one pound, cloves two ounces, nutmegs, ginger, and carraway ſeeds, each four ounces; coriander ſeeds four ounces, diſtil them in a ſtill with a worm, put it into a veſſel, and add to it Spaniſh liquorice
bruiſed,

bruised, raisins of the sun stoned, of each two pounds; cinnamon four ounces; dates, stoned and the white skin taken off, four ounces. if you intend it to be yellow, put in two ounces of saffron, five pounds of white or brown sugar-candy. keep it close nine or ten days, stir it once a day, and, if you would have it green, leave out the saffron, and add either angelica or green corn sufficient to give it a fine colour; a week after, put in three grains of ambergrease and musk; after standing ten days, put a flannel into a a large sieve, set the sieve under a funnel, and strain it into the cask; let it stand till it is fine, bottle it off, and the older you keep it, the better

Wormwood water

Take the outward rinds of a pound and a half of lemons, one pound of orange peels, tops of dried wormwood, and winter cinnamon, of each half a pound, flowers of camomile four ounces, little carcamums not husked, cloves, cubebs, and camels hay, of each one ounce; cinnamon, nutmegs, carraway seeds, each two ounces, spirits of wine six quarts, spring water four gallons and a half, infuse all these together three or four days, distil them in a Balneo Mariæ, and it will prove an excellent stomachic cordial.

Simple wormwood water.

Take one pound of dried wormwood, four ounces of carraway seeds bruised, and three gallons of spirits of wine; infuse and distil them in one pound and a half of sugar, and bottle it for use

Snail water.

Take comfry and succory roots, of each four ounces, liquorice three ounces, leaves of harts tongue, plaintain ground-ivy, red nettles, yarrow, brookline, water-cresses, dandelion, and agrimony, of each two large handfuls, gather the herbs in dry weather,
do

do not wash them, but wipe them with a clean cloth; then take five hundred snails cleaned from their shells, but not scoured; a pint of the whites of eggs beat up to a water; four nutmegs grosly beat, and the yellow rind of one lemon and one orange, bruise all the roots and herbs, and put them with the other ingredients in a gallon of new milk, and a pint of Canary wine; let them stand close covered eight and forty hours; distil them in a common still over a gentle fire; it will keep good a year, and must be made at spring or autumn, for three months only stop the bottles with paper, then cork them, when you use this water, put an equal quantity of milk

To make cheap mead.

Take the honey out and add as much water to the honeycombs as they will sweeten, let it stand to be well mixed, boil it well, and scum it, when an egg will swim at the top, it will be sufficiently boiled, then put it into a wooden vessel, let it stand till cold, and bottle it in stone bottles; you may boil it either with lemon, thyme, rosemary, or cowslips

How to make common mead.

Take a gallon of honey, eight gallons of water, a quarter of a pound of ginger sliced, and six whites of eggs beat with the shells, put all these into a convenient vessel to boil, and let them boil till a fourth part of the liquor be wasted, scumming it all the time, to each gallon of water, put a handful of rosemary; when your liquor is sufficiently boiled, put in the remainder of your ingredients, and when all is boiled, strain your liquor through a hair sieve, and let it stand till it is thoroughly cold; then put a pint of ale yeast to the vessel, then put in the liquor, and if the weather is cold, let it stand two or three days before you bottle it.

Frontiniac

Frontiniac mead.

Fifty pounds of honey, fifty pounds of Belvedera raisins, fifty gallons of water, boil these about fifteen minutes, keeping it well scummed; pour it into the working tub, and put into it a pint of ale yeast, letting it work till the yeast begins to fall; when taken clear off, tun it, with the raisins, and throw into the cask a quart of white elder flowers; take care to attend it in change of weather, let it continue in the cask twelve months, and then fine it down with wine fining, and bottle it off.

A fourth sort of mead.

To each gallon of water take a pound and a half of honey, boil them with an handful of sweet marjoram, sweet bryer, and bay leaves, with a sprig of rosemary, a few nutmegs quartered, mace, cloves, and cinnamon; tie the spices up in a cloth, boil all together a full hour, and scum it all the time, when boiled, put it into a pale or other wood vessel proportionable, and work it with about a spoonful of yeast to each gallon; turn it when it works to the top, and when fine bottle it; a week after you have bottled it, if you find it not clear, rack it, and let it stand three or four days longer.

To make cyder or perry as clear as rock water.

Take two quarts of cyder, half a pint of milk, and put them both in an Hippocrates's bag; when it looks clear bottle it up, and in one month it will be fine, sparkle, and ripe for drinking.

How to make a most excellent wine, called Briton's wine.

Take currants both red and white, gooseberries red and green, mulberries, rasberries, and strawberries of different sorts, cherries of different sorts, but none of
the

the little black ones; grapes, black and white; all the fruit must be thoroughly ripe, and take an equal quantity of each, throw them into a mash-tub, and bruise them lightly, take golden pippins, and norpareils, chop and bruise them well, and mix them with the others; to every two gallons of fruit, put one gallon of spring water; boil all twice a day for a fortnight, then press it through an hair bag into another vessel, and have ready a wine hogshead; put into the hogshead one hundred raisins of the sun with their stalks, fill it with the strained juice, lay the bung on lightly, and when it has quite done hissing and working, put in one gallon of right French brandy, and stop the vessel close; let it stand six months, then peg it, and see if it be fine, and if it is, bottle it; if it be not fine, stop it up for six months longer, and then bottle it; the longer it is kept the better it will be, and it is necessary you put in half a dozen bay leaves along with your French brandy

You may alter the flavour of your wine by different sorts of raisins, as Belvedera, Sumerner, Malaga, or with the raisins of the sun.

Note: When you have drawn off the wine, throw the raisins into a still, and that will produce you fine brandy

Raisin wine

First get a good white-wine cask, and in every hogshead put in two hundred weight of raisins with their stalks on; fill it up with water, let it stand till it has done working, and put to it two quarts of French or raisin brandy, when it has quite done working, stop it up, and let it stand six months; then peg it, and if it proves fine, bottle it, then take the lees distil them, and they will produce you a fine brandy, or you may make fine vinegar of the lees Malaga raisins make a sweet wine; raisins of the sun a dry wine; Belvedera raisins make fine cape wine; and each having a different flavour.

Elder

Elder wine.

When the elders are pretty ripe take the berries from the stalks, put them in a jug, stop it close, and and set it in a kettle of water; after it has boiled an hour strain your juice, and to every pint of juice add half a pound of fine sugar boiled to a thin syrup; and to every gallon of raisin wine, made as above, put a pint of the syrup; let it stand till it is fine, and bottle it if your raisin wine is ready

To give your raisin wine different flavours.

Put into your cask a few walnut leaves; into your sweet wine a few bay leaves, just to give a flavour; and to another a few elder flowers

To make them like red port

Take twelve gallons of black wine, two gallons of French brandy, the rest raisin wine, this will serve for a hogshead

To make it like Madeira wine.

Take a walnut, peel off the outside, chop the walnut and steep it in half a pint of red wine, then pour it to a bottle of the dry wine, and so proportionably to a greater quantity,

To make an excellent grape wine.

Take ripe grapes gathered on a clear day, put them in a fine canvas, and gently press them so as not to break the stones; strain the liquor well, let it settle in a cask, and draw off the clear liquor into a well seasoned vessel, stop it close for forty-eight hours, and give it vent by boring a hole at the top of the cask, and stopping it occasionally with a peg, in two or three days stop it close, and it will be fit for drinking in a quarter of a year, and not before, and will prove but very little inferior to your best French wine. To season

son your vessel use scalding hot water, and dry it with a rag dipped in brimstone, and fix it to the bung-hole with the cork.

English malmsey

Take of English galengal and cloves each one drachm, beat them to powder, infuse them a day and a night in a pint of aquavitæ in a wooden vessel kept close covered, put it into good claret, and it will make twelve or fourteen gallons of good malmsey in five or six days, the drugs may be hung in a bag in the vessel.

To make grape wine

When ever your vines are well grown so as to bring full clusters, be careful to disencumber them of some part of their leaves that too much shade the grapes, but so that the sun may not too swiftly draw away the moisture and wither them; stay not till they are all full ripe, for then some will be over ripe, some burst, some rot; but every two or three days pluck off the ripest grapes, and place them in a shady place to dry, not too thick, lest they contract a heat thereby and grow musty, so do from day to day, till you have got a sufficient quantity; then put them into an open vessel, and gently press them, taking care not to break the stones, since you will thereby hurt the wine by making it bitter.

Note In foreign countries it is usual to press down the grapes with the feet, or with a wooden trencher; but I always use my hands for that purpose, as being the more decent way.

Having thus bruised the grapes to a mash, and a tap placed at the bottom of your cask, tie a hair cloth over the faucet, and set it running; take out the pulp, and gradually press it in a side-press till the liquor is sufficiently drained; then, having a new vessel well seasoned and aired, with a lighted rag, dipped in brimstone, burn it till it becomes dry; pour the liquor in through a sieve funnel to stop the dregs, and put a pebble at the bung-hole, that thereby it may ferment

and

and clear itself; after it has thus stood for ten or twelve days, draw it gently off into another cask, well seasoned, that the lees may remain in the first, stop this as before, and when it has passed over its ferment, which you may tell by its calmness, and the pleasantness of its taste, cover it up; and in this manner of your ordinary white grapes you may make a good white wine; of the red, a good claret; and if your claret wants colour, then you may heighten it with a little brazil boiled in about a quart of it, and strained very clear; the white grapes, if not too ripe, give a good rhenish taste, and are wonderfully cooling; and a sort of Muskadel grapes produce a curious sweet wine, little inferior to Canary, and altogether as pleasant and wholsome, so that with a small charge, labour, and industry, we might well furnish ourselves with what we are beholden to strangers for, at a much greater expence, besides their unwholsomeness to the English constitution.

Cowslip wine.

Boil eight gallons of water and twelve pounds of sugar one hour, scum them, and take them from the fire; pour into the liquor one peck of cowslips well picked, and let them stand till luke warm, afterwards put in the juice of twelve or fourteen lemons, with some peel to lie in while it stands covered with a cloth, which must be four days; strain off the liquor, press the juice from the cowslips, and mix all together; after which, let it stand twenty-one days in a great glass bottle, and, when clear, bottle it up.

To make wine of quinces.

Clean your quinces with a coarse cloth, grate them with a grater, press them thro' a linen strainer, and afterwards through a flannel, to every gallon of liquor put three pounds of double-refined sugar, and when it is melted, pour it off as long as there is a settlement at the bottom; continue melting and clearing of it for twenty-four hours, and then put it in a vessel; let it stand a week, and bung it up, if it has done working;
you

you then may either draw it off in bottles, or let it be put into another vessel, and kept for use

To make Morello cherry wine.

Let cherries be very ripe, pick off the stalks, and bruise the fruit without breaking the stones, put them in an open vessel together, let them stand twenty-four hours, and press them, to every gallon put two pounds of fine sugar, put it in your vessel, and when it has done working stop it close; let it stand three or four months, then bottle it, and in two months it will be fit for drink.

To make apricot wine.

Take three pounds of sugar and three pounds of water, let them boil together, and be well scummed, put in six pounds of apricots pared and stoned, let them boil till they are tender, take them off, and, when the liquor is cold, bottle it up, you may, if you please, after you have taken out the apricots, let the liquor boil very little with a sprig of flowered clary in it; the apricots make very good marmalade and are very good for present spending

To make damson wine.

Gather your damsons, dry and weigh them, and bruise them with your hand; put them into an earthen stein that hath a faucet, and to every eight pounds of fruit put a gallon of water; boil your water, scum it, and put it to your fruit scalding hot; let it stand two whole days, draw it off into a vessel fit for it, and to every gallon of liquor put two pounds and a half of fine sugar; let the vessel be full, stop it close, and the longer it stands the better, it will keep a year, the small damson is best, and when you bottle it off you may put a small lump of fine sugar to every one

To make birch wine

In March bore a hole in a tree and fix a faucet in the hole, and it will run three days without hurting the tree; then stop the hole with a peg, and the next year draw off the same quantity; put to every gallon of the liquor a quart of good honey, stir it well, boil it an hour, scum it, and put in a few cloves and a piece of lemon peel; when it is almost cold, put to it so much ale yeast as to make it work like new ale, let it work six weeks or more, and bottle it off, it will be fit to drink in a month's time, and will keep good a year or two; you may use sugar instead of honey, the quantity of two pounds to every gallon, or something more if you intend to keep it long; this is a very wholsome as well as pleasant liquor; an opener of obstructions, good against the phthisic and the spleen, as also the scurvy, and the stone, it will abate heat in a fever, and hath been given with good success.

To make sage wine.

Boil twenty-six quarts of spring water a quarter of an hour, and when it is blood-warm, put twenty-five pounds of Malaga raisins picked, rubbed, and shred; add to it half a bushel of red sage finely shred, and a porringer of ale yeast; stir all well together, and let it stand in a tub for six or seven days, close covered, stirring it well once a day; then strain it out, and put it in a rundlet, let it work three or four days, stop it up, and, after standing six or seven days, put in a quart or two of fine Malaga sack, and when fine, bottle it off.

N B All other fruit wine you may make according to the different receipts above described.

Bitter wine.

Take two quarts of strong white wine, infuse in it one drachm of rhubarb, a drachm and a half of gentian root, Roman wormwood, tops of carduus, centaury, camomile flowers, of each three drachms; yellow

low peel of oranges, half an ounce of nutmegs, mace, and cloves, of each one drachm, infuse all for forty-eight hours, strain it, and drink a glass an hour before dinner

How to rack wine.

This is done with such instruments as are useful and appropriated to the manner of doing it, and cannot be so well described as by seeing it done, however, observe this, let it be done then when the wind is full north, and the weather clear and temperate, that the air may the better agree with the constitution of the wine, and may make it take more kindly, as it is proper to be done in the increase of the moon

To make wines scent well, and give them a curious flavour.

Take powders of sulphur two ounces, and half an ounce of calamus; incorporate them well together, put them into a pint and half of burrage water, and let them steep therein a considerable time, draw off the water, and melt the sulphur and calamus in an iron pan, and dip in as many rags as will soak it up; put the rags into a cask, rack off the wine, put in a pint of rose water, and stop up the hogshead, roll it up and down for half an hour, and then let it continue still two days; by ordering it thus, any red or Gascoigne wine will have a pleasant scent and taste

To keep wine from souring.

Boil a gallon of wine with some beaten oister shells and crabs claws calcined, strain out the liquid part, and when it is cool put it into the wine of the same sort, and it will give a pleasant lively taste; a stone of unflaked lime will also keep your wine from souring

Milk punch.

Take two quarts of water, one quart of milk, half a pint of lemon juice, and a quart of brandy, sugar it to your taste, put the milk and water together a little warm, then add the sugar and lemon juice, and stir together, put in the brandy, and run it through a flour bag till it is fine, you may bottle it, and it will keep a fortnight or more.

Milk punch for present drinking.

To two quarts of water put two quarts of French brandy, a dozen and a half of lemons, three quarters of a pound of double-refined sugar, and three pints of new milk, strain it frequently through a jelly-bag, till it is clear and fine; you must make it two or three days before you use it, and may bottle it off, but it will preserve its goodness for a time.

Quince wine

Clean the quinces with a coarse cloth, then grate them, and press them through a linen strainer to clear them from the gross thickness, and then through a flour strainer, to every gallon of this liquor put two pounds of single-refined sugar, let it settle, and pour it off, this do several times till there is no sediment; then pour it into your vessel, and let it remain unstopped six days, then keep it six months, and bottle it off, if it is fine, if not, pour it into another

Note. You must observe, as an unexceptionable rule, that all English wines must be kept in cool cellars

Birch wine, as made in Sussex.

Take the sap of birch fresh drawn, boil it as long as any scum rises, and to every gallon of liquor put two pounds of good sugar; boil it half an hour, scum it clean, and when almost cold, set it with a little yeast spread on a toast, and let it stand five or six days in an open vessel, stirring it often, then take a barrel exactly big enough to hold the liquor, burn in a lighted match, and stop in the smoak; shake out the ashes, and pour in a pint of sack or rhenish, working it well about, pour in your wine, stop it close for six months, and if it be perfectly fine you may then bottle it off

Black

Black cherry wine.

Boil six gallons of spring water one hour, bruise twenty-four pounds of black cherries, but not to break the stones, and pour the water boiling hot over them, stir the cherries well in the water, and let them stand twenty-four hours, strain off the liquor, and to every gallon put two pounds of good sugar, and let it stand a day longer, pour it off clean into your vessel, stop it close, and when it is very fine draw it off into your bottles.

Red cherry wine, as made in Kent.

When your cherries are full ripe, strip off the stalks and stamp them, as apples, till the stones are broke, put the mash into a tub, cover it up close for three days, put and press it in a cyder-press, and let the liquor run into a tub; let it stand covered for three days, take off the scum very carefully for fear of its breaking, and pour it into another tub to clear it of the lees; let it stand two days more, scum it, and if your cherries are sweet, put only one pound and a half of sugar to each gallon of liquor, stir it well together, cover it close, and let it rest till the next day; pour it carefully off the lees, let it rest another day, and then pour it into the vessel in which you design to keep it; bung it up, keep it seven or eight months, and, if fine, bottle it off, if it be not fine, draw it off into another vessel to fine. This wine, if made agreeable to these my well experienced directions, will keep a year in bottles.

How to improve cyder, and make it perfectly fine.

When it is first made, put six ounces of stone brimstone into a hogshead, to give it a colour, put a gallon of good French brandy, highly tinctured with cochineal, beat one pound of alum, and three pounds of sugar-candy, and put them to it when you stop it up; when it is fine bottle it, and it will be perfectly good.

How

CONFECTIONER. 119

How to make beer, wine, or any other liquors fine.

Set your vessel on two boards the length of the barrel, lay upon them a large quantity of bay salt, and fix the barrel on the salt, let it thus stand a fortnight, and it will be perfectly fine, this certainly clears the liquor preferable to isingglass, and is much neater, being only put to the outside of the vessel; it ought at all times to be observed, that all liquors whatever ought to be fined before they begin to fret, or they will never be good.

Compound parsley water.

Take parsley roots four ounces, fresh horse-raddish root, and juniper berries, of each three ounces; the tops of St John's wort, biting arsmart, and elder flowers, of each two ounces; the seeds of wild carrots, sweet fennel, and parsley, of each one ounce and a half, mix these ingredients together, bruise them, and add thereto two gallons of French brandy, and two gallons of soft water; let them steep in the still three or four days, and draw it off. this is an excellent remedy for the gravel

Compound horse-raddish water

Take the leaves of the two sorts of scurvy-grass, fresh gathered in the spring, of each six ounces, add four ounces of brooklime and water-cresses, and of horse-radish two pounds, of fresh arum-root six ounces, winter bark and nutmeg, of each four ounces, dried lemon peel two ounces, and of French brandy two quarts, and draw all off by distillation, this water is good in both dropsical and scorbutic ales

Compound piony water

Take eighteen piony roots fresh gathered, six ounces of bitter almonds, the leaves of rosemary, rue, and thyme, and flowers of lavender dried, of each

three

three ounces; of cinnamon, cubebs, seeds of angelica, coriander seed, carraway and annifeeds, each half an ounce; one gallon of rectified spirits of wine, with five gallons of soft water, and draw off three gallons by distillation. This is good in all nervous disorders.

Compound scordium water.

Take of citrons, sorrel, goats rue, and scordium, of each one pound, and London treacle two ounces; distil them in an alembick, with two quarts of spirits of wine, and a sufficient quantity of water; of this you may draw off one gallon.

Annifeed water.

Take twelve ounces of annifeeds, three gallons of proof spirits, one gallon and a half of spring water, infuse them all night in a still, and with a gentle heat draw off what runs smooth and clear, sweeten it with two pounds of brown sugar, and if you would have it very fine, distil it again, and add some more annifeeds.

Carraway water.

Take three gallons of proof spirits, and of water half a gallon; add to them half a pound of carraway seeds bruised, distil and sweeten the juice with a pound and half of brown sugar.

Cardamum water.

Take carraway seeds, coriander seeds, pimento, and lemon peel, of each four ounces; mix them with three gallons of proof spirits, a gallon and a half of spring water, distil them, and sweeten the water with one pound and a half of sugar.

The three foregoing waters are each of them very cheap, and a most wholsome cordial.

Strong

Strong palsey water.

Take the spirits of five gallons of the best old sherry sack, distilled in an alembick, add to it cowslip flowers, the flowers of burrage and buglofs, and of the lilies of the valley, each a handful, also rosemary flowers, sage, and betony flowers, the same quantity; these must all be procured in their season, and put into some of the spirits aforesaid, in an open mouthed quart glass; let them remain in the spirits till you are ready to distil the waters, and carefully stopped up, take lavender flowers in their season, strip them from their stalks, and fill a gallon glass with them, pour to them the remainder of your spirits, and cork them close as before; let them be in the sun six weeks, and put these and the rest of the flowers in the two glasses, then add balm, motherwort, spike flowers, bay-leaves, and orange leaves, of each half an ounce; cut and put them to the former flowers and spirits, and distil them together in an alembick, and make three runnings of it, first a quart glass, which will be exceeding strong; then a pint glass, which will be almost as good, and then a third pint, or as much as will run, for when it runs weak, which you know by its taste and the colour, being whiter, you will have drawn about that quantity; mix your runnings together, and take citron, or the yellow rind of a lemon peel, six drachms of spice seeds, and of cinnamon one ounce, with nutmegs, mace, cardamums, and yellow saunders, of each half an ounce; of lignum aloes one drachm, make these into a gross powder, adding a few jujubs that are fresh, stoned, and cut small. put these ingredients into a large sarsnet bag, and hang it in the water as aforesaid, take two drachms of prepared pearls, of ambergrease, musk, and saffron, one scruple each; red roses dried one ounce, these may be put in a bag by themselves, and hang in the spirits as the other, close it well, that no air gets in, and let it rest six weeks; take out the water, prefs the bags dry, and keep the water in narrow mouthed glaffes, and ftop it up

The ufe of this water.

It is fo ftrong and powerful that it cannot be taken without the affiftance of fome other thing, but when dropt on crumbs of bread and fugar, you muft take it the firft thing in the morning, at four in the afternoon, and the laft thing at night, you muft not eat for an hour either before or after you take it, it is exceeding efficacious in all fwoonings, weaknefs of heart, decayed fpirits, palfies, apoplexies, and both to help and prevent a fit; it will alfo deftroy all heavinefs and coldnefs in the liver, reftores loft appetite, and fortifies and furprifingly ftrengthens the ftomach

The fecond water, to be made on the ingredients of the firft.

When the firft water has run what is ftrong, there will remain a fmaller fort at the bottom of the alembick, take and prefs the herbs and flowers, and put them into a gallon and a half of the beft fherry, and let them ftand clofe ftopt five weeks; diftil them, and let the liquor run as long as it remains ftrong, pour it into a glafs where the farfnet bags are, and let them be in this fecond liquor fix weeks, clofe ftopped, then you may ufe it as the former

Note: This is to bathe any part affected with weaknefs.

Syrup of rofes.

Take a gallon of foft water, put it into an earthen pan, and throw in as many rofe leaves as will foak it up; cover them clofe, fet them on a flow fire, and when they begin to fimmer take them from the fire, and let them ftand till next day, ftrain them, fet the liquor on the fire, and when it boils, put in as many rofe buds as will foak it up; let it ftand till the next day, and ftrain it off again; repeat this, day after day, till there is not above pint and a half of water

left,

left, put this into a long pipkin, proper to make your syrup in, set it on the fire, when it boils put in a pound and a half of sugar, scum it, let it boil, and when it is cold, bottle and keep it for use.

Syrup of colts-foot.

Take of colts-foot six ounces, maiden hair two ounces, hyssop one ounce, liquorice-root one ounce, boil them in two quarts of spring water, till one fourth is consumed, then strain it, and put to the liquor two pounds of fine powder sugar; clarify it with the whites of eggs, and boil it till it is nearly as thick as honey.

Balsamic syrup of Tolu

Take six drachms of the balsam of Tolu, and boil it to twenty ounces of spring water, till the half is consumed, taking care not to scum them, then add twenty ounces of the best refined sugar, make it to a syrup without further boiling, and when it is cold strain it off

Syrup of Tolu

Boil half an ounce of pearl barley in three several waters, strain off the last water, and when it is settled, take three pints of it, and two ounces of Tolu; let it simmer till almost a pint is wasted, and put in two pounds of loaf sugar, boiling it gently to a syrup to what thickness you please, and when almost cold strain it

Syrup of mulberries

Take the clear juice of mulberries, to each quart of clear juice, put one pound of white sugar, and make it into a syrup over a slow fire

Syrup of poppies.

Take two pounds of corn poppy-flowers, and four pounds of warm spring water, let them stand to infuse twenty-four hours, then strain them, and add fresh flowers to the water, letting the water be warm when you put them in, let them stand close covered till next day, strain it off, and with an equal quantity of sugar, boil it to a syrup.

Syrup of violets.

Take one pound of fresh pickled violets, boil five half pints of soft water, and pour it over the violets; let it stand close covered in a well glazed earthen vessel for twenty-four hours, and dissolve in it twice its own weight of white sugar, so as to make a syrup without boiling.

Syrup of clove jilly-flowers.

Gather the flowers early in the morning, pick them clean, and cut the white from the red, to a quart of flowers put two quarts of spring water, let it stand for two days in a cold place, and after boil it till it come to a quart; strain it off, and put in half a pound of double-refined sugar, and boil it up again for three or four minutes, pour it into a china bowl, let it stand to cool, and when it is quite cold scum it, put it into bottles, cork them well, and tie them down with leather.

Syrup of buckthorn.

Gather your berries in the heat of the day, and set them in an earthen pot into the oven, then squeeze out the juice, and put the juice of one peck of berries to two pounds of Lisbon sugar, and boil them together a quarter of an hour, then let it cool, and bottle it.

Syrup for a cough or asthma.

Take a handful of unset hyssop, a handful of coltsfoot flowers, a handful of black maiden hair, and two handfuls of white horse hound, boil these in three quarts of water, and when half is boiled away, take it off, and let the herbs stand in it till they are quite cold, squeeze the herbs very dry, strain the liquor, and boil it a quarter of an hour, scum it well, and to every pint put in half a pound of white sugar, and boil it, when it becomes a syrup, put it to cool, and bottle it off, do not cork the bottles, but tie papers over them; this is an exceeding fine syrup for a cough, by taking a spoonful both night and morning, and one whenever the cough is troublesome.

A second syrup

Take one ounce of conserve of roses, one ounce of brown sugar candy, and two of raisins of the sun, cleared of their stones; to these add some flower of brimstone, mix them together, and take a spoonful night and morning

Syrup of Balsam

Put an ounce of balsam of Tolu into a quart of spring water, and boil them two hours; put in a pound of white sugar-candy finely beat, and boil it half an hour longer, take out the balsam, strain the syrup twice through a flannel bag, and when it is cold bottle it, this syrup is excellent for a cough, by taking a spoonful at night, and a little whenever your cough is troublesome.

Barley syrup.

Take a pound of fresh barley, put it in water, and when it boils throw the water away; so do a second water, put to the barley a third water, the quantity of six quarts, and boil it while one third is consumed, strain out the barley, and put to the water a handful of scabious, tormentil, hyssop, agrimony, hare-hound, maiden-hair, sanicle, and betony, burage, bugloss, rosemary, marygolds, sage, violets, cowslips, of these a pint each when picked, a pound of raisins of the sun stoned; half a pound of figs cut; a quarter of a pound of dates stoned, and the white skin next the stone taken off, half a pound of green liquorice, carraway seeds, fennel seeds, and anniseeds, of each one ounce, hartshorn, ivy, elecampane roots, of each one ounce, fennel roots, asparagus roots, couch-grass roots, polypodium roots, oak-parsley roots, of each one handful; after they are cleaned, bruise the liquorice and seeds, and slice your roots; put the aforenamed ingredients into your barley water, let them boil very softly, close covered twelve hours, afterwards strain it, and press the juice from the ingredients, and let it stand twenty-four hours; take the liquor off clear, and add to it half a pint of damask-rose water, and half a pint of hyssop water, with a pint of the juice of colts-foot clarified; a drachm of saffron, three pints of the best virgin honey, and as many pounds of sugar as there are quarts of liquor; boil this an hour and a half, keeping it clean scumed, then bottle it, cork it well, and preserve it for your own proper use

Note. This syrup is good for an old cough; and three spoonfuls, night and morning, mixed with the same quantity of wine or sack, is sufficient to take

A second way to make syrup of violets

Pick the violets from the greens, and sift them clean; then to every four ounces of violets add half a pint of water, and one pound of coarse sugar, first take the water and put into it half the sugar; set it over the fire, clarify and scum it well, stamp your violets in a marble mortar, and when they are well beat, infuse them in the clarified syrup for some time, minding

minding the syrup is not too hot when you put in the violets, when they have infused a while strain them, and preserve some of the juice in another vessel, and let it stand by; put in the rest of the sugar, set it again on the fire, scum it, and keep it stirring; when it hath boiled softly some time, put in the rest of the juice, and one drop of the juice of lemon, set it once more, for a small time on the fire, and when cold, put it up for use.

Syrup of marsh-mallows

Take of the fresh roots of marsh-mallows two ounces, and parsley roots one ounce; liquorice root, the tops of marsh-mallows and mallows, and figs, of each half an ounce, raisins stoned two ounces, sweet almonds blanched one ounce, let all these steep one day in three quarts of clear barley-water, and boil it to two quarts, press out the decoction, and when grown fine by standing in the liquor, dissolve one ounce of gum-arabic, and four pounds of fine sugar, and make it into a syrup

Another way

Take four ounces of marsh-mallow roots, grafs-roots, asparagus-roots, liquorice, raisins stoned, of each half an ounce, the tops of marsh-mallows, pellitory, pimpernel, saxifras, plantain, maiden-hair, white and black, of each one handful, red sisars, one ounce of each, bruise all these, and boil them in three quarts of water, till they come to two; then put to it four pounds of white sugar to make it a syrup, and clarify every pint with the white of an egg, or isinglass

Syrup of saffron.

Take a pint of balm water and a pint of the best Canary, half an ounce of English saffron; open the saffron, and put it into liquor to infuse, and let it stand close covered, so as to be hot and not boil, and continue so for twelve hours; then strain it out as hot as you can, and add to it three pounds of double-refined sugar, and boil it till it is well incorporated; when cold bottle it; a spoonful, in any simple water or wine, is a high cordial.

Syrup of buckthorn.

Take three quarts of the clarified juice of buckthorn berries, four pounds of brown sugar, make them into a syrup over a gentle fire, and, while it is warm mix it with a drachm of the distilled oil of cloves dissolved on a lump of sugar, for it will not dissolve in the syrup.

Note: Take great care you have the true buckthorn, as there are many spurious ones; they may be known by the number of seeds; the genuine buckthorn having four, the alder buckthorn has only two, and the cherry buckthorn one only.

Another syrup for a cough, or asthma.

Take pennyroyal and hyssop water, of each half a pint, slice to them a small stick of liquorice and a few raisins of the sun stoned; let them simmer a quarter of an hour, and make it into a syrup with brown sugar-candy, boil it a little, and then put in four or five spoonfuls of snail-water, and give it a second boil, when it is cold, bottle it, and take a spoonful morning and night, with three drops of balsam of sulphur put into it.

Another, and a valuable one.

Take a handful of maiden-hair, a handful of oak-lungs, and a handful of fresh moss; boil these in three pints of spring water, till it comes to a quart, strain it out, and put to it six pennyworth of saffron tied up in a rag, adding thereto a pound of brown sugar-candy, boil the liquor up to a syrup, and when cold bottle it.

Note:

Note You may take a spoonful of this syrup, as often as you find your cough troublesome

There are many more syrups, but too many for this book, but these mentioned are the most choice ones, not only in themselves, but as the directions in them contained, are an invariable guide to the lady in the other various kinds of syrups

To make conserve of hips

Gather your hips before they grow soft, cut off the heads and stalks, slit them in half, and take out all the seed and white; put them in an earthen pan, stir them every day, left they grow mouldy, and let them stand till they are soft enough to rub through a coarse hair sieve; they are a dry berry, and rub through with some difficulty, add to them their weight in sugar, and mix them well together without boiling, keeping it in gallypots for use

Conserve of red-roses.

Take red-rose buds, bruise them in a marble mortar, adding by degrees fine powder sugar sifted, to the quantity of three pounds; beat them till no particles arise, and till the whole becomes a firm and solid mixture

Conserve of orange peel

Take the clear rind of oranges, steep them in water of a moderate heat till they are tender, then strain the water from them, pound them in a marble mortar, and strain them through a sieve; then bring the pulp to a proper consistence over a gentle fire, and add to it thrice its quantity of sugar, and let it be reduced into a conserve by beating it in a mortar

Conserve of quince

Pare the quince, take out the cores and seeds, then cut them into small pieces, boil them till they are soft, to eight pounds of quince put in six pounds of sugar, boil them to a consistence.

To make rob of elder

Take a peck of elderberries and bake them in an earthen pan, squeeze the juice out, and put it in a silver or tin stew-pan, then set it on a gentle fire, it will be three days stewing; you must stir it often, and when you see it so thick that you may cut it with a knife, it is enough, then put it in gallypots for use, whilst it is hot.

To make spirit of clary

Take a gallon of good sack, a pint of the juice of clary, a pound of clary-flowers, as many clove-jilly-flowers, and half as many arch-angel-flowers, as many comfry-flowers, and as many flowers of lilies of the valley, let these steep in the sack all night, then put it into a glass still, the softer it distils, the stronger 'twill be; you must take great care to keep in the spirit, by pasting the still every where, let it drop through a bag of good ambergrease, upon as much sifted white sugar-candy as you think will sweeten it, 'tis a very high cordial.

To make spirit of carraways.

To a quart of true spirits of sack, put two pounds of good smooth sugared carraways, bruise them, and put them into a bottle, with a grain of the best ambergrease, pour the spirit on them, and seal the cork very close, set it in the sun for a month, strain 't off and keep it always close stopt for use.

Cordial of black cherry water

Take two quarts of strong claret, and four pounds of black-cherries full ripe, stamp them, and put them to the wine, with one handful of angelica, one handful of balm, and as much cardmus, helt as much mint, and as many rosemary flowers as you can hold in both your hands; three handfuls of clove-jilly-flowers, two ounces of cinnamon cut small, one ounce of nutmegs, put all these into a deep pot, let them be well stirred together, then cover it so close that no air can get in, let it stand one day and a night then put it into your still, which you must also paste close, and draw off as much as runs good, sweeten it with sugar-candy to your taste

A very rich cherry cordial

Take a stone pot that has a broad bottom, and a narrow top, and lay a row of black cherries and a row of very fine powdered sugar, do this till your pot is full, measure your pot, and for every gallon it holds, put a quarter of a pint of true spirit of wine, you are to pick your cherries clean from soil and stalks, but not wash them; when you have thus filled your pot, stop it with a cork, and tie first a bladder, then a leather over it; and if you fear it is not close enough, pitch it down close, and then bury it in the earth six months, or longer, then strain it out, and keep it close stopped for your use, it will revive when all other cordials fail.

The following receipts were sent to the author, when the book was just printed, by a good housekeeper

To make rhubarb tarts.

Take stalks of English rhubarb, that grow in the gardens, peel and cut it to the size of gooseberries; sweeten it, and make them as you do gooseberry tarts: how to make the crust, you have in the Art of Cookery

These tarts may be thought very odd, but they are very fine ones, and have a pretty flavour; the leaves of rhubarb are a fine thing to eat for a pain in the stomach, the roots for tincture, and the stalks for tarts

Angelica

Angelica tarts.

Take the stalks, peel them, cut them into little pieces, pare some golden pippins or non-pareils, of each an equal quantity, first take away the parings of the apples, and the cores, boil them in as much water as will cover them, with a little lemon peel and fine sugar, till it is like a very thin syrup, then strain it off, and set the syrup on the fire again with the angelica, let it boil about ten minutes, then when the crust is ready, lay a sliced apple and a layer of angelica, so on, till the patty pans are full, and bake them, filling them first with the syrup

To preserve damsons, or bullace

Put your damsons in a pot, to two quarts of water, put a pound of fine sugar, and bake them in a slow oven two hours, then set them in a cool place a week, and pour over them as much rendered beef suet as will be an inch thick, it must be put on hot every time you take any out; and they will keep all the year.

Another way to do them

Make a syrup of water and sugar, gather the fruit before they are ripe, and put them into the cold syrup; then set them on a slow fire, and keep them stirring gently round, till they are a little coddled, but not broke; put all into a pot that has a little mouth, and when cold, pour on more, till it is an inch thick on the top, and set it by

To make anniseed biscuits.

To every twelve pounds of dough, put twenty ounces of butter, a pound of sugar, two ounces of anniseeds, with a little rose-water, and what spice you think fit, and bake it in a moderate oven

To keep gooseberries.

Gather them on a very fine day, when full grown, before they are ripe, pick them, have ready nice clean bottles, fill them to the neck, then cork them, and rosin the top of the bottle that no air can get into it, then set them in a kettle of water, up to the neck, over a slow fire; when the water is scalding hot, take out the bottles, and the next day dig a hole in the earth, and put your bottles in; cover them up with the earth again, and keep them for winter, some keep them only in a dry place, but the earth keeps them better.

A very rich almond-cream, called steeple-cream.

Make a very strong jelly of hartshorn, and that it may be so, put half a pound of good hartshorn to five pints of water; let it boil away near half; strain it off through a jelly-bag; then have ready, beaten to a very fine powder, six ounces of almonds which must be carefully beat up with one spoonful of orange-flower water, with six or eight spoonfuls of very thick cream then take near as much cream as you have jelly, and put both into a skillet, and strain in your almonds, sweeten it to your taste with double-refined sugar, set it over the fire, and stir it with care constantly, 'till 'tis ready to boil, so take it off, and keep it stirring 'till it is near cold; then pour it into narrow-bottom'd drinking-glasses, in which let it stand a whole day; when you would turn it out, put your glasses into warm water for a minute, and it will turn out like a sugar-loaf.

To make orange-posset

Squeeze the juice of two Seville oranges and one lemon into a china bason, that holds about a quart, sweeten this juice with the syrup of double-refined sugar, put to it two spoonfuls of orange-flower water, and strain it through a fine sieve, boil a large pint of cream,

cream, with some of the orange peel cut thin; when it is pretty cool, pour it into a bason of juice through a flannel, which must be held as high as you can from the bason, it must stand a day before you use it, when it goes to table, stick slips of candied orange, lemon, and citron peel on the top.

To make black caps, the best way

Take a dozen and a half very large French pippins, or golden rennets, cut them in half and lay them with the flat side downwards, lay them as close to each other as you can, press the juice of a lemon into two spoonfuls of orange-flower water, and mix them all together; shred some lemon peel into it, and grate some double-refined sugar over it; put them into a quick oven, and half an hour's baking will be sufficient.

To make Newport cream cheese.

You must get a vat made a quarter and a half high, the bottom nor top must not be fastened, and it must be made four square, with holes all over them; then take two quarts of good thick cream, two quarts of stroakings, and a gallon of new milk, and set it with rennet, as for common cheese, when it is come, take out the curd with a China saucer, and put it into the vat, strewing a little clean dry salt thereon, fill up the vat, till all the cheese is in, press it as other cheese, let it stand in the vat two or three days, till all is out, and turned often while it is in; salt it two days, when you take it out you must let it dry without rubbing, and make it in May: if you desire it exactly four square, let the vat be full a quarter and a half high, and the square want an inch of a quarter.

To make a pretty sort of flummery.

Put three large handfuls of oatmeal ground small into two quarts of fair water, let it steep a day and night, then pour off the clear water, and put the same quantity of fresh water to it; strain it through a fine hair sieve,

sieve, and boil it till it is as thick as hasty pudding; stir it all the while, that it may be extremely smooth, and when you first strain it, before you set it on the fire, put in one spoonful of sugar, and two of good orange flower water; when it is boiled enough, pour it into shallow dishes for your use

To make cracknels

To a quart of flour take a pound of butter, half a nutmeg grated, the yolks of four eggs beat, with four spoonfuls of rose water, put the nutmegs and eggs into the flour, and wet it into stiff paste, with cold water, then rowl in the batter and make them into shape; put them into a kettle of boiling water, when they swim, take them out with a skimmer, and throw them into cold water; when they are hardened lay them out to dry, and bake them on tin plates

Right Dutch wafers.

Take four eggs, and beat them very well; then take a good spoonful of fine sugar, one nutmeg grated, a pint of cream, and a pound of flour, a pound of butter melted, two or three spoonfuls of rose water, and two good spoonfuls of yeast; mix all well together, and bake them in your wafer-tongs on the fire, or in an oven

The Nun's biscuit.

Take the whites of six eggs, and beat them to a froth, take also half a pound of almonds, blanch and beat them with the froth of the whites of your eggs as it rises, then take the yolks with a pound of fine sugar, beat these well together, and mix your almonds with your eggs and sugar; then put in a quarter of a pound of flour, with the peel of two lemons grated, and some citron finely shred, bake them in little cake pans in a quick oven, and when they are coloured turn them on tins to harden the bottoms, but before you set them in the oven again, strew some double-refined sugar on them finely sifted, remember to butter your pans, and fill them but half full.

To make oil of eggs

Take eight large eggs, and new laid, boil them hard, then take the yolks out, be careful not to put any white of the eggs in, and break them small, and let them stand to be cold; then have a quick fire ready, and put them in an iron ladle, with a bit of hogs lard, the bigness of a walnut; you must stir it with a stick cut flat at the end, and when it begins to melt, keep stirring as fast as you possibly can, in a moment before it turns to oil, it will dry, you must have a cup ready to pour it in as fast as you see a drop of oil come, with that quantity of eggs you will have a tea cup of oil, if you stir quick, if not, you will not see a drop of oil.

To make tumbles

To a pound of fine flour, a pound of double-refined sugar, and two ounces of coriander seeds, the yolks of two eggs, and wet it stiff with a little rose water; then rowl them out the bigness of your finger, and make them in the form of a figure of eight, then put them on tins and bake them in a slow oven, watch them all the time, about ten minutes will bake them.

To make currant shrub

Take white currants full ripe, mash them with your hands, then strain them through a hair sieve, and to one gallon of rum or brandy, put five pints of the currant juice, and a pound of lump sugar; cover it up close, and let it stand two or three days, stirring it twice a day, then run it through a jelly bag it is best to put half the spirits to the juice, and add the other half when you bottle it off

To preserve beet roots.

Boil your beet roots for four hours, till you see it quite soft; then make a syrup of a pint of spring water and half a pound of sugar, and boil the beet root in it, for a quarter of an hour; then put it in gallypots for use When you want to use them for sauce, soak them in warm water for ten minutes or more, and slice them into oil and vinegar.

To dry artichoaks red.

Boil your artichoaks in water till you see they are soft, then take them out, and pound some cochineal very fine, and mix in fresh water, and boil them again a quarter of an hour, then dry them in bags for a quarter of an hour.

To preserve apples red all the year.

Get a dozen of pippins or pearmanes, pare them, put a quart of water to them, one pennyworth of cinnamon stick, grate part of a lemon rind, and some cochineal steeped in water, half a pound of loaf sugar, then send them to the oven, tie over them a paper and after that coarse paste, don't forget to scoop a hole in the middle of the apples to let the liquor thro' them, let them stand in a slow oven, when you think they are enough, take them out of the oven, take off the paper, and let them stand in the syrup; in the morning drain it from them, and put to it a little water, a pound, or a pound and a half of sugar, as you would have a quantity of syrup for them, and when you have scum'd them well, clear it with the white of an egg, when that is done put in your apples again, and let them boil in the syrup till it be clear; then put in as much cochineal as will make them of a good colour, sometimes take the apples out lest they should break, and let the syrup be boiling and scum it often; when your apples are half enough, let them stand in the syrup all night, and in the morning set it over the fire, which must be of charcoal; let it boil up, then take the apples out, and put them in again, when your syrup is boiled to a thickness for keeping, and your apples a good colour, shred your lemon peel, and put in a half an ounce of candid orange cut in thin slices; put your apples into the pot you design to keep them in, and when your syrup is half cold put it on your apples, and put them up for use.

To pickle colliflowers red

Get the best you can, let your water boil with a little salt in it, then put in your colliflowers, the faster it boils the whiter it will be, do not let it be too much done, then let it cool, and prepare your pickle; for red, you must take allegar, salt, and some of your colouring, and spice in it, if you would have them white, take white wine vinegar, salt and spices, having the white of your colliflower, your pickle being cool, you put them into it keeping them for use.

To pickle turnips

Pare and cut them in slices, put them into spring water, and let them boil a little while, but not too much, take them out and cut them into what form you please; then put them into alegar and salt for some days, then take them out and wipe the pickle from them, boil the alegar and some of your colouring with spices, and when they are cold put them together, and keep them for use.

To make violet drops

Take an ounce of violets and cut the whites from the leaves, and prick them very well, a quarter of a pound of sugar, as much water as will make a candy, when your candy is ready, put in your flowers, and let them just have a boil, then drop them on paper and they will grow hard soon.

To get mildew out of linen

Scrape some chalk, and mix it pretty thick with water, dip the cloth in it, and hang it in the sun to dry, repeat this till it is out.

To make clove-jilly-flower wine.

To every gallon of water add two pounds and a half of sugar, boil it half an hour, scum it well, and
pour

pour it boiling hot upon the flowers, picked all from the stalks, let it stand till cold; then put in four or five spoonfuls of yeast; or according to the quantity you make. let it stand three days, stir it every twelve hours; when you barrel it, strain it through a flannel, stop it close and bottle it in three weeks; put into every bottle a clove and a bit of sugar; don't cork it close for some time

To pickle carrots.

Take them of a middle size, the yellowest you can get, half boil them, and cut them in what shape you please, and let them lie to cool; then take as much vinegar as will cover them, boil a pennyworth of saffron in a bit of muslin, with a little salt; when your pickle is cold put them into a pot, cover them up close, let them stand all night, then pour out the pickle, and boil it with Jamaica pepper, mace, cloves, and salt; when cold, pour it on the carrots, and keep it for use.

To keep walnuts all the year moist.

Gather your nuts in a very dry day, and take care they don't lye on the ground to be bruised; as you gather them, put them into a deep earthen pot, when full, cover them with a paper, and then with a leather, and over that a wet bladder; set them in a dry place

THE COMPLEAT BILLS OF FARE

SEVERAL families have desired I would in my Book of Confectionary, give them a few bills of fare of little deserts, fit for private families, but as it is a thing depends entirely on fancy, and indeed, what they have to set it out with, and the season of the year for fruits, &c. I am at some loss how to give directions in writing; but as it may be a little guide to the young and unexperienced, I have given them in the best manner I can, agreeable to the method they are now set out, ice cream is a thing used in all deserts, as it is to be had both winter and summer, and what in London is always to be had at the confectioners.

Giving directions for a grand desert would be needless, for those persons who give such grand deserts, either keep a proper person, or have them of a confectioner, who not only has every thing wanted, but every ornament to adorn it with, without giving any trouble to the family, when supposed to be taken up with other affairs; though every young lady ought to know both how to make all kinds of confectionary and dress out a desert; in former days, it was looked on as a great perfection in a young lady to understand all these things, if it was only to give directions to her servants, and our dames of old, did not think it any disgrace to understand cookery and confectionary.

But for country ladies it is a pretty amusement, both to make the sweetmeats and dress out a desert, as it depends wholly on fancy, and but little expence.

	Lemon Cream.	
Peaches		Plumbs
	A large dish with figures and grass or moss about it, and flowers only for shew.	
Plain ice cream.		Rasberry cream
Apricots.		Nectarines
	Syllabubs.	Peaches

CONFECTIONER.

<table>
<tr><td></td><td>Peaches in Brandy.</td><td></td></tr>
<tr><td>Colour'd wafers.</td><td></td><td>Heart biscuit.</td></tr>
<tr><td>Compote of pears.</td><td>A dish or salver, a dish of jellies, intermixed with wet sweat-meats.</td><td>Compote of chesnuts.</td></tr>
<tr><td>Savoy biscuit.</td><td></td><td>White wafers.</td></tr>
<tr><td></td><td>Morello cherries in brandy.</td><td></td></tr>
</table>

<table>
<tr><td></td><td>A ghizzard cream.</td><td></td></tr>
<tr><td>Lemon cream in glasses.</td><td></td><td>Colour'd sweat-meats in glasses.</td></tr>
<tr><td>Ratafia drops.</td><td>High flowers, images, &c. dress'd with grass, moss, and other ornaments according to fancy.</td><td>Spunge biscuits.</td></tr>
<tr><td>Wet sweet-meats in glasses.</td><td></td><td>Jellies.</td></tr>
<tr><td></td><td>A floating island.</td><td></td></tr>
</table>

The

142 THE COMPLEAT

The above middle frame should be made either in three parts or five, all to join together, which may serve on different occasions, on which suppose gravel walks, hedges, and variety of different things, as a little Chinese temple for the middle, or any other pretty ornament; which ornaments are to be bought at the confectioners, and will serve year after year, the top, bottom and sides are to be set out with such things as are to be got, or the season of the year will allow, as fruits, nuts of all kinds, creams, jellies, whip syllabubs, biscuits, &c &c and as many plates as you please, according to the size of the table

All this depends wholly on a little experience, and a good fancy to ornament in a pretty manner, you must have artificial flowers of all sorts, and some natural out of a garden in summer time do very well intermixed

As gizzard cream is not in the fore part of the book, I shall give it here · take the skins of three large gizzards of fowl or turkey; put them into a quart of cream, sweeten it and spice it as you like, boil all together, then strain it into your dish, and it will be fine and thick.

	Lemon cream.	
Peaches.		Plumb.
Plain ice cream.	A dish only for shew, with figures, &c. &c.	Rasberry cream
Apricots.		Nectarines
	Syllabubs.	

	Ice cream.	
Fruit		Fruit.
	One large dish in the middle of jellies, cream, and Syllabubs.	
Fruit.		ruit.
	Ice cream of different sorts.	

	Jellies and biscuits.	
Dry'd apples.		Chesnuts.
	Sweet meats wet and dry.	
Almonds and rasins.		Stew'd pears.
	Jellies and biscuits.	

	Stew'd pippins with thick cream poured over them:	
Pot oranges.		Postatia nuts.
	Wet and dry sweet meats, and jellies both red and white, intermix'd, adorn'd with flowers.	
Ice cream.		Ice cream.
Walnuts.		Ratafia cakes.
	Pears stew'd purple with fine ratafia cream, pour'd over them.	

Ice

144 THE COMPLEAT

Ice cream

Fruit.		Fruit.
	Two salvers one above another, whip'd syllabubs and jellies intermix'd with crisp'd almonds, and little ratafia cakes, one little one above all, with preserv'd orange or pine apples, little bottles with flowers to adorn it, and knicknacks strew'd about the salver.	
Creams.		Little cakes.
Fruit.		Fruit.
Large Seville oranges sliced with double refined sugar strew'd over.		Almonds and raisins.

Ice cream, different colours.

Ice cream.

Stew'd pippins.		Little pot oranges.
Compote of pears	A Grand Trifle.	Compote of chesnuts
Postatia nuts		Nonpareil

Ice creams, different colours.

Jellies.

CONFECTIONER

Jellies.

Fruit.		Fruit.
Almond hedgehogs.	A high salver with syllabubs, a little rais'd above with a preserved orange or lemon.	Almond creams.
Fruit.		Fruit.

Jellies.

Whip'd syllabubs.

Bloomage, stuck with Almonds.		Ice cream.
Chesnuts.	Two salvers one above another, on the bottom one jellies, the top a large glass cup cover'd with rasberry cream.	Dry'd cherries.
Ice cream.		Almond flummery.

Whip'd syllabubs.

As to all sorts of little biscuits, almonds, knicknacks, &c. &c. on the middle of the salver, or wet sweet-meats in little glasses; you intermix them according as you fancy.

H Whip'd

146   THE COMPLEAT

	Whip'd syllabubs.	
Golden pippins.		Filberts.
	Jellies, lemon cream, and sweet-meats both wet and dry, piled upon salvers with crisp'd almonds, and knicknacks.	Large oranges slic'd and sugar strew'd over
Chesnuts.		
Plumbs.		Nonpareils
Bloomage.		Ice cream
	Whip'd syllabubs.	

	Lemon cream.	
Dry'd cherries.		Dry'd plumbs
Winter pears		Grapes
	Jellies	
Postalia nuts		Almonds and raisins.
	Almond flummery.	

	Jellies.	
Peaches.		Nectarine
Filberts.		Green gages.
	Whip'd syllabubs.	
Creams.		Almond flummery
Cherries.		Walnuts
Fine pears.		Grapes.
	Jellies.	Ice

CONFECTIONER 147

	Ice cream.	
Filberts		Dry'd plumbs.
	Floating island.	
Grapes.		Pears.
Nonpareils.		Walnuts.
	Ice cream different colours.	

	Ice cream, different colours.	
	Whip'd syllabubs.	
Clear jellies.		Lemon cream in glasses.
Nonpareils.	In the middle a high pyramid of one salver above another, the bottom one large, the next smaller, the top one less; these salvers are to be fill'd with all kinds of wet and dry sweet-meats in glass, baskets or little plates, colour'd jellies, creams, &c biscuits, crisp'd almonds and little knicknacks, and bottles of flowers prettily intermix'd, the little top salver must have a large preserv'd Fruit in it.	Golden pippins.
Bloomage stuck with almonds.		Bloomage stuck with almonds.
Pottaha nuts.		Almonds and raisins.
Lemon cream in glasses.		Clear jellies in glasses.
	Whip'd syllabubs. Ice cream, different colours.	Lemon

H 2

Lemon cream, in glasses.

| Peaches. | | Nectarines. |

Ice cream.

Walnuts.

| Grapes. | | Golden pippins. |

| Almond flummery stuck with almonds. | Two large salvers in the middle, one above another, in the top whip'd syllabubs, a garland of flowers rais'd above them, the bottom one fill'd with clear jellies. | Almond flummery stuck with almonds. |

Filberts.

| Nonpareils. | | Pears. |

Ice cream.

| Apricots. | | Plumbs. |

Lemon cream, in glasses.

Note: You are to alter the side plates as you think proper, or with such fruit and things as you can get

CONFECTIONER 149

<table>
<tr><td></td><td>Whip'd syllabubs.</td><td></td></tr>
<tr><td>Filberts.</td><td></td><td>Ratafia cakes.</td></tr>
<tr><td>Plies</td><td>A large dish of fruit of all sorts, piled up, and set out with green leaves</td><td>Jellies.</td></tr>
<tr><td>Ratafia cakes.</td><td></td><td>Filberts.</td></tr>
<tr><td></td><td>Whip'd syllabubs.</td><td></td></tr>
</table>

<table>
<tr><td></td><td>Raberrice cream.</td><td></td></tr>
<tr><td>Walnuts.</td><td></td><td>Nonpareils.</td></tr>
<tr><td>Green grapes, and black.</td><td>Jellies piled up on two salvers, a large glass in the middle.</td><td>Black grapes, and green.</td></tr>
<tr><td>Pears.</td><td></td><td>Filberts.</td></tr>
<tr><td></td><td>Gooseberry fool.</td><td></td></tr>
</table>

<table>
<tr><td></td><td>Peaches and Nectarines.</td><td></td></tr>
<tr><td>Walnuts.</td><td></td><td>Plumbs.</td></tr>
<tr><td>Grapes</td><td>Jellies, and cream intermix'd.</td><td>Grapes.</td></tr>
<tr><td>Currants.</td><td></td><td>Filberts.</td></tr>
<tr><td></td><td>Peaches and Nectarines.</td><td>Rasberries.</td></tr>
</table>

H 3

150 THE COMPLEAT

     Rasberries.

Filberts.   Gooseberries

Sugar   Small biscuits

Red cherries.   Two salvers,   Black cherries.
     one above an-
     ther, on the
     top cream, in a
Small   large glass bowl,
biscuits   the bottom   Sugar
     jellies.

Currants.   Filberts

     Strawberries.

     Almond flummery,
     stuck with almonds.

Sugar   Potato
in plates.   pies

     One large sal-
     ver in the
     middle fill'd
Almond   with jellies and   Small
cream in   whip'd syllabubs,   cheesecakes
cups.   and a garland of
     flowers meeting
     a lover

Ratafia   Sugar
cakes.   in plates

     A bason of cream.

To keep walnuts all the year

Take your walnuts full ripe, and peel them; then dry them well in the sun for a week or more, rub them often with a cloth till you see no mould on them, then keep them in a bag, in a dry place, and when you want any for a desert, crack and peel them quite clean, but take care that you keep the nut whole, or in quarters, then put them in some spring water, warm as you may bear your finger in, let them stand three or four hours, then shift them in cold spring water, and let them stand all night, the next day, when you go to set your desert put them in glasses, and they will be crisp and fine as when fresh gathered

To make oil of filberts

Take the large Barcelona filberts, crack them, heat a pair of tongs red hot, and hold the kernel in them over a cup, and out of one nut you will have three or four drops of oil, heat your tongs every time you take a fresh nut, and with a pint of nuts you will have half a small tea-cup full of oil.

To make oil of paper.

Take a sheet of strong writing-paper, and roll it cross ways, roll a large pin in the corner for the oil to drop out, set the top a fire, and hold it over a cup, and there will come out three or four drops

Compound of oils for family uses, are made of oil of olives, and other simples, herbs, flowers, roots, &c

The way of making them is thus, having bruised your herbs or flowers, you would make your oil of, put them in an earthen pot, and to two or three handfuls of them pour on a pint of oil, cover the pot with paper, set it in the sun about a fortnight or less, according as the sun is in hotness, then having warmed it very well by the fire, take out the herbs and press them very hard, adding the oil that comes out to the other in the pot, put in as many more herbs, set them in the sun as before, the oftener you repeat this, the stronger your oil will be at last when you conceive it strong enough, boil both herbs and oil together, I mean, the last herbs, till the juice be consumed, which you will know by its leaving its blushing, and the herbs will be crisp, then strain it whilst it is hot, and keep it in a stone bottle, or a glass vessel for use

To make syrup of water cresses

Take a peck of water cresses, bruise them a little put two quarts of water to them, and let them stand twenty-four hours; boil them up for a little while, then squeeze them, and put in a pound of the finest sugar you can get, and boil it together till it comes to a quart, be careful not to boil it in a copper saucepan, and when it is cold put in half a pint of good rum, and bottle it for use

To make a syrup of nettles

Take a quantity of nettles and pound them, and squeeze them through a cloth to a pint of juice add half a pound of Lisbon sugar and boil it half an hour; then cool it and bottle it off

To keep green peas all the year

Gather your peas young, and on a very fine dry day; when the water boils put in your peas, give them two or three boils and drain them, then throw them on a cloth till quite dry, have ready clean bottles, fill them up to the neck; then pour in some beef suet, cork the bottles, tye them down with a bladder and a leather, and dig a hole in the earth, put them in, and cover them till Christmas; and when you want to use them, let your water boil, put in a piece of butter, and some coarse sugar.

To keep kidney beans.

Gather them of a dry day, dry them in the sun, and keep them in papers, in a dry place, and before you use them, lay them in warm water.

To make ice.

Put in a pail of water, one ounce of sal armoniac, and it will all turn to ice, but if the salts are not right it will not do.

To make eau de luce

Oil of amber one ounce, high rectified spirit of wine four pounds; put them into a bottle and let them stand four or five days, shaking the bottle often; then put into this spirit four pounds of the choicest amber, finely powdered, and let it digest three days, then you will have a rich tincture of amber fit for use

That being made, take sixteen pounds of strongest spirit of sal armoniac, and add to it the above tincture, with eight pounds of high rectified spirit of wine.

How to use the ordinary still

You must lay the plate, then wood-ashes thick at the bottom; then the iron pan, which you are to fill with your ingredients and liquor, then put on the head of the still, make a pretty brisk fire, till the still begins to drop, then slacken it so as just to have enough to keep the still at work, mind all the time to keep a wet cloth all over the head of the still to keep in the steam thereof, and always observe not to let the still work longer then the liquor is good, and take great care you do not burn the still; and thus you may distil what you please, if you draw the still too far, it will burn, and give your liquor a bad taste.

To make plague water

Roots.	Flowers	Seeds
Angelica,	Wormwood,	Hart's-tongue,
Dragon,	Suckery,	Whorehound,
Maywort,	Hysop,	Fennel,
Mint,	Agrimony,	Mellilot,
Rue,	Fennel,	St John-wort,
Carduus,	Cowslips,	Comfry,
Origany,	Poppies,	Featherfew,
Winter-savoury,	Plantain,	Red rose-leaves,
Broad thyme,	Setfoyl,	Wood-forrel,
Rosemary,	Bugloss,	Pellitory of the wall,
Pimpernell,	Vocvain,	Heart's-ease,
Sage,	Maidenhair,	Centaury,
Fumetory,	Motherwort,	Seadrink, a good handful of each of the above-mentioned thing
Coltsfoot,	Cowage,	Gentian-root,
Scabeous,	Golden-rod,	Dock-root,
Burridge,	Gromwell,	Butter-bur-root
Saxafreg,	Dill.	Piony-root,
Bitony,		Bay-berries,
Liverworth,		Juniper-berries of each of these a pound
Germander		

One ounce of nutmegs, once ounce of cloves, and half an ounce of mace, pick the herbs, and flowers, and shred them a little Cut the roots, bruise the berries, and pound the spices fine; take a peck of green walnuts, and chop them small, mix all these together, and lay them to steep in sack-lees, or any white-wine lees, if not, in good spirits, but wine-lees are best Let them lie a week, or better be sure to stir them once a day with a stick, and keep them close covered, then still them in an alembick with a slow fire, and take care your still does not burn. The first, second, and third running is good, and some of the fourth. Let them stand to be cold, then put them together

To make surfeit water

You must take scurvy-grass, brook-lime, water-cresses, roman wormwood, rue, mint, balm, sage, clivers, of each one handful; green merery two handfuls, poppies, if fresh, half a peck, if dry a quarter of a peck, cochineal six-pennyworth, saffron six-pennyworth, anniseeds, carraway-seeds, coriander-seeds, cardamon-seeds, of each an ounce, liquorice two ounces scraped, figs split a pound, raisins of the sun stoned a pound, juniper-berries an ounce bruised, nutmeg an ounce beat, mace an ounce bruised, fennel-seeds an ounce bruised, a few flowers of rosemary, marygolds and sage-flowers, put all these into a large stone jar, and put to them three gallons of French brandy, cover it close, let it stand near the fire for three weeks. Stir it three times a week, and be sure to keep it close stopped, and then strain it off, bottle your liquor, and pour on the ingredients a gallon more of French brandy. Let it stand a week, stirring it once a day, then distil it in a cold still, and this will make fine white surfeit water.

You may make this water at any time of the year, if you live at London, because the ingredients are always to be had, either green or dry; but it is the best made in summer.

Of the proper season for distilling.

Flowers of all kinds must be distilled in their proper seasons. To begin with the violet. Its colour and smell can only be extracted when it is in its greatest vigour, which is not at its first appearance, nor when it begins to decay. April is the month in which it is in the greatest perfection, the season being never so forward

forward in March, as to give the violet its whole fragrancy.

The same must be observed of all other flowers. And let them be gathered at the warmest time of the day, the odour and fragrancy of flowers being then in their greatest perfection.

The same observation holds good with regard to fruits; to which must be added, that they are the finest, and of the most beautiful colour, especially those from whence tinctures are drawn; they must be free from all defects, as the goods would by that means be greatly detrimented.

Berries and aromatics may be distilled at any season, all that is necessary being a good choice. But in this distillers are sometimes mistaken, as may easily happen without a very accurate knowledge.

Of sugar spirit.

I mean by a sugar-spirit, that extracted from the washings, scumings, dross, and waste of a sugar baker's refining-house.

These recrementitious, or drossy parts of the sugar are to be diluted with water, fermented in the same manner as melasses or wash, and then distilled in the common method. And if the operation be carefully performed, and the spirit well rectified, it may be mixed with foreign brandies, and even arrack in a large proportion, to great advantage; for this spirit will be found superior to that extracted from treacle, and consequently more proper for these uses.

Of raisin-spirit.

By raisin spirit, I understand, that extracted from raisins, after a proper fermentation.

In order to extract this spirit, the raisins must be infused in a proper quantity of water, and fermented in the manner described. When the fermentation is completed, the whole is to be thrown into the still, and

and the spirit extracted by a strong fire, so you see the raisins out of a cask, after the wine is made to do.

The reason why we here direct a strong fire, is, because by that means a greater quantity of the essential oil will come over the helm with the spirit, which will render it much fitter for the distiller's purpose; for this spirit is generally used to mix with common malt goods, and it is surprising how far it will go in this respect, ten gallons of it being often sufficient to give a determining flavour, and agreeable vinosity to a whole piece of malt spirits.

It is therefore well worth the distiller's while to endeavour at improving the common method of extracting spirits from raisins, and perhaps the following hint may merit attention.

When the fermentation is completed, and the still charged with fermented liquor, as above directed, let the whole be drawn off with as brisk fire as possible, but instead of the cask or cann, generally used by our English distillers for a receiver, let a large glass, be placed under the nose of the worm, and the receiver applied to the spout of the separating-glass, by this means the essential oil will swim upon the top of the spirit, or rather low wine, in the separating-glass, and may be easily preserved at the end of the operation.

The use of this limpid essential oil is well known to distillers, for in this resides the whole flavour, and consequently may be used to the greatest advantage, in giving that distinguishing taste and true vinosity, to the common malt-spirits.

After the oil is separated from the low wine, the liquor may be rectified in Balneum Mariæ into a pure and almost tasteless spirit, and therefore well adapted to make the finest compound cordials, or to imitate or mix with the finest French Brandies, arracks, &c.

In the same manner a spirit may be obtained from cyder. But as its particular flavour is not so desirable as that obtained from raisins, it should be distill'd in a more gentle manner, and carefully rectified in the common manner, of rectification; by which means a

very

very pure and almost insipid spirit will be obtained, which may be used to very great advantage in imitating the best brandies of France, or in making the finest compound waters or cordials.

Of the distilling of simple waters by the alembic

The plants designed for this operation are to be gathered when their leaves are at full growth, and a little before the flowers appear, or, at least, before the seed comes on, because the virtue of the simple expected in these waters is often little, after the seed or fruit is formed, at which time plants begin to languish the morning is best to gather them in, because the volatile parts are then condensed by the coldness of the night, and kept in by the tenacity of the dew not yet exhaled by the sun

This is to be understood, when the virtue of the distilled water resides principally in the leaves of plants, as it does in mint, marjoram, pennyroyal, rue, and many more but the case differs when the aromatic virtue is only found in the flowers, as in roses, lilies of the valley, &c in which case we chuse their flowery parts, whilst they smell the sweetest, and gather them before they are quite opened, or begin to shed, the morning dew still hanging on them

In other plants the seeds are to be preferred, as in anise, caraway, cumin, &c where the herb and the flower are indolent, and the whole resides in the seed alone, where it manifests itself by its remarkable fragrance, and aromatic taste We find that seeds are more fully possessed of this virtue, when they are at perfect maturity

We must not omit that that these desirable properties are found only in the roots of certain plants appears in avens and in orpine, whose roots smell like a rose Roots of this kind should be gathered for the present purpose, at that time when they are richest in these virtues; which is generally at that season of the year just before the begin to sprout, when they are to be dug up in a morning

If the virtues here required be contained in the barks or woods of vegetables, then these parts must be chosen for that purpose.

The subject being chosen, let it be bruised, or cut, if there be occasion, and with it fill two thirds of a still, leaving a third part of it empty, without squeezing the matter close; then pour as much rain or river water into the still as will fill it to the same height; that is, two thirds together with the plant. fit on the head, luting the juncture, so that no vapour may pass though, and also lute the nose of the still-head to the worm. Apply a receiver to the bottom of the worm, that no vapour may fly off in the distillation; but that all the vapour being condensed in the worm, by cold water in the worm-tub, may be collected in the receiver.

Let the plant remain thus in the still to digest for twenty-four hours, with a small degree of heat. Afterwards raise the fire, so as to make the water in the still boil, which may be known by a certain hissing noise, proceeding from the breaking bubbles of the boiling matter; as also by the pipe of the still-head, or the upper-end of the worm, becoming too hot to be handled, or the smoaking of the water in the worm-tub heated by the top of the worm; and lastly, by the following of one drop immediately after another, from the nose of the worm, so as to form an almost continual stream. By all these signs we know the requisite heat is given; if it be less than a gentle ebullition, the virtues of the simple, here expected, will not be raised. on the contrary, when the fire is too strong the water hastily rises into the still-head, and fouls both the worm and the distilled liquor; and the plant being also raised, it blocks up the worm; for which reason it is no bad caution to fasten a piece of fine linen before the pipe of the still head; that, in case of this accident, the plant may be kept from stopping up the worm. but notwithstanding this precaution, if the fire be too fierce, the plant will stop up the pipe of the still-head, and, consequently, the rising vapour finding no passage, will blow off the still head, and throw the boiling liquor about the

still-

still-house, so as to do a great deal of mischief, and even suffocate the operator, without a proper caution, and the more oily, tenacious, gummy, or resinous the subject is, the greater the danger, in case of this accident, because the liquor is the more frothy and explosive.

Let the due degree of fire therefore be carefully observed and equally kept up, as long as the water, distilling into the receiver, is white, thick, odorous, sapid, frothy and turbid; for this water must be carefully kept separate from that which follows it. The receiver, therefore, should be often changed, that the operator may be certain that nothing but this first water comes over; for there afterwards arises water that is transparent, thin, and without the peculiar taste and flavour of the plant, but generally somewhat tartarous and limpid, though somewhat obscured and fouled by white dreggy matter; and if the head of the still be of copper, and not tinned, the acidity of this last water corrodes the copper, so as to become green, nauseous, emetic and poisonous to those who use it, especially to children, and persons of weak constitutions.

The first water above-described, principally contains the oil and presiding spirit of the plant; for the fire by boiling the subject, dissolves its oil, and reduces it into small particles, which are carried upwards by the assistance of the water, along with those parts of the plant that becomes volatile with their motion. And, if the vessels are exactly closed, all these being united together, will be discharged without loss, and without much alteration, into the receiver; and, consequently, furnish us with a water richly impregnated with the smell, taste, and particular virtues of the volatile parts of the plants it was extracted from.

The water of the second running, wants the volatile part above described, and has scarce any other virtue than that of cooling.

And this is the best method of preparing simple waters, provided the two sorts be not mixed together, for both of them would be spoiled by such a mixture.

Hence

Hence it plainly appears at what time, with the same degree of fire, quite contrary virtues may arise from a plant; for so long as a milk water continues to come over from such plants as are aromatic, so long the water remains warming and attenuating; but when it comes to be thin and pellucid, it is acid and cooling.

Hence we may also learn the true foundation for conducting of distillation; for if the operation be stopped, as soon as ever the white water ceases to come over, the preparation will be valuable and perfect; but if, through a desire of increasing that quantity, more be drawn off, and the latter acid part suffered to mix with the first running, the whole will be spoiled, or at least rendered greatly inferior to what it would otherwise have been.

Such is the general method of procuring simple waters, that shall contain the volatile virtues of the plants distilled; some rules are however necessary to render it applicable to all sorts of plants, these rules are the following.

1 Let the aromatic, balsamic, oily, and strong-smelling plants, which long retain their natural fragrance, such as balm, hyssop, juniper, marjoram, mint, origanum, pennyroyal, rosemary, lavender, sage, &c. be gently dried a little in the shade; then digest them, in the same manner as already mentioned, for twenty-four hours, in a close vessel, with a small degree of heat, and afterwards distil in the manner above delivered, and thus they will afford excellent waters.

2 When waters are to be drawn from barks, roots, seeds, or woods that are very dense, ponderous, tough and resinous, let them be digested for three, four, or more weeks, with a greater degree of heat, in a close vessel, with a proper quantity of salt added, to open and prepare them the better for distillation. The quantity of sea-salt is here added, partly to open the subject the more, but chiefly to prevent putrefaction, which otherwise would certainly happen in so long a time, and with such a heat as is necessary in this case, and

and so destroy the smell, taste, and virtues expected from the process.

3 Those plants which diffuse their odour to some distance from them, and thus soon lose it, should immediately be distilled after after being gathered in a proper season, without any previous digestion, thus borage, bugloss, jessamin, white lilies, lilies of the valley, roses, &c are hurt by heat, digestion, or lying in the air. All these may be done in a common still, but they won't be too strong

Of the method of procuring a simple water from vegetables, by previously fermenting the vegetable before distillation

By this elegant method we obtain the virtues of plants very little altered from what they naturally are, though rendered much more penetrating and volatile. The operation is performed in the following manner.

Take a sufficient quantity of any recent plant, cut it, and bruise it if necessary; put it into a cask leaving a space empty at top of about four inches deep, then take as much water as would, when added, fill the cask of the same height, including the plant, and mix therein about an eighth part of honey, if it be cold winter weather; or a twelfth part, if it be warm. In the summer the like quantity of coarse, unrefined sugar might be added instead of honey, or half an ounce of yeast to each pint of water will have the same effect, though most prefer honey for this purpose. When the proper quantity of honey is added to the water, let it be warmed and poured into the cask, and set into a warm place to ferment for two or three days, but the herb must not be suffered to fall to the bottom, nor the fermentation above half finished. The vice must then be immediately committed to the still, and the fire raised by degrees, for the liquor, containing much fermenting spirit, easily rarifies with the fire, froths, swells, and therefore becomes very subject to boil over, we ought therefore to work slower, especially at first.

By this method there will come over at first, a limpid, unctuous, penetrating, odorous, sapid liquor, which is to be kept separate: after this there follows a milky, opaque, turbid liquor, still containing something of the same taste and odour; and at length comes one that is thin, acid, without either smell, or scarce any property of the plant.

The first water, or rather spirit, may be kept several years, in a close vessel, without changing or growing ropy. It also excellently retains the taste and odour of the plant, though a little altered; but if less honey were added, less heat employed, or the fermentation continued for a smaller time, the distilled liquor of the first running would be white, thick, opaque, unctuous, frothy, and perfectly retain the scent and taste of the plant, or much less altered than in the former case; though the water will not be sharp and penetrating. After this is drawn off a tartish, limpid, inodorous liquor will come over.

And thus may simple waters be made fit for long keeping without spoiling, the proportion of inflammable spirit, generated in the fermentation, serving excellently to preserve them.

Of the simple waters commonly in use.

Simple waters are not so much used at present as they were formerly, and perhaps one reason for their being neglected, is the bad method used in distilling them; the process is carried on in the same manner with every herb; though some should be gently dried, and others distilled green; some should be drawn with the cold, and others with the hot still.

The general rule that should be observed with regard to the hot still is, that all herbs should have twice their weight of water added to them in the still, and not above a fourth or a sixth part of it drawn off again; for simple waters have their faints, if drawn too low, as well as those that are spirituous.

Some plants, particularly balm, require to have the water drawn from them cohobated, or poured several times on a fresh parcel of the herb, in order to give it a proper degree of strength or richness. Others, on the contrary, abound too much with an essential oil that floats on the diftilled water, in this cafe all the oil fhould be carefully taken off. Laftly, thofe that contain a more fixed oil, fhould be imperfectly fermented, in the manner laid down, before they are diftilled; of this kind are caduus, camomile, &c.

The fimple waters now commonly made, are orange-flower-water, rofe-water, cinnamon, fennel-water, pepper-mint-water, fpear-mint-water, balm-water, pennyroyal-water, Jamaica pepper-water, caftor-water, fimple water of orange-peel, and of dill feed.

Of orange-flower-water

Some degree of attention is requifite to draw a fimple and odoriferous water from the orange-flowers, the fire muft be carefully regulated, for too fmall a degree will not bring over the effential oil of the flowers, in which their odoriferous flavour confifts and, on the contrary, too ftrong a fire deftroys the fragrancy of the water, and is very apt to fcorch the flowers, and give the water an empyreumatic fmell. Care fhould alfo be taken to faften the receiver to the end of the worm with a bladder, to prevent the volatile parts from evaporating. The quantity of water, alfo, fhould be carefully attended to, if you hope to fucceed in the operation. The following receipts will anfwer the intention.

Receipt for orange-flower-water

Take twelve pounds of orange-flowers, and twenty-four quarts of water and draw over three pints. Or, take twelve pounds of orange-flowers, and fixteen quarts of water; draw over fifteen quarts, carefully obferving what has been obferved at the beginning with regard to the regulation of the fire.

Of pepper-mint-water

Pepper-mint is a very celebrated ftomachic, and on that account greatly ufed at prefent, and its fimple water often called for.

Receipt

Receipt for a gallon of pepper-mint-water

Take of the leaves of dried pepper-mint, one pound and a half, water two gallons and a half, put all into an alembick, and draw off one gallon, with a gentle fire.

The water obtained from pepper-mint, by distillation in Balneum Mariæ, is more fragrant, and more fully impregnated with the virtues of the plant than that drawn by the alembick. The same may be said with regard to that extracted by the cold still; when the cold still is used, the plant must be green, and if possible committed to the still with morning dew upon it.

Of spear mint-water

Spear-mint is also, like pepper-mint, a stomachic, and therefore constantly used.

Receipt for one gallon of spear mint-water

Take the leaves of dried spearmint, one pound and a half, water two gallons and a half, put all into an alembick, and draw off one gallon, by a gentle fire.

This water, like that drawn from pepper-mint, will be more fragrant if distilled in Balneum Mariæ, or the cold still, but if the latter be used, the same caution must be observed of distilling the plant green.

Receipt for a gallon of Jamaica pepper-water.

Take of Jamaica-pepper half a pound, water two gallons and a half, draw of one gallon, with a pretty brisk fire. The oil of this fruit is very ponderous, and therefore this water is best made in an alembick.

It is a very noble aromatic, and deserves to be used more frequently than it is at present. The simple water drawn from it is a better carminative than any other simple water at present in use.

Of lemon-water

The peel of the lemon, the part used in making this water, is a very grateful bitter aromatic, and on that account, very serviceable in repairing and strengthening the stomach

Receipt for ten gallons of lemon-water.

Take of dried lemon-peel four pounds, clean proof spirit ten gallons and a half, and one gallon of water Draw off ten gallons by a gentle fire Some dulcify lemon water, but by that means its virtues as a stomachic, are greatly impaired.

Receipt for ten gallons of compound angelica-water

Take of the roots and seeds of angelica, and of sweet fennel-seeds, of each one pound and an half, of the dried leaves of balm and sage, of each one pound; slice the roots, and bruise the seed and herbs, and add to them of cinnamon one ounce, of cloves, cubebs, galangals, and mace, of each three quarters of an ounce, of nutmegs, the lesser cardamom seed, pimento, and saffron, of each half an ounce, infuse all these in twelve gallons of clean proof spirit, and draw off ten gallons, with a pretty brisk fire It may be dulcified or not, at pleasure

This is an excellent composition, and a powerful carminative, and good in all flatulent cholics, and other griping pains in the bowels It is also good in nauseas, and other disorders of the stomach

It may not be amiss to observe here, that in distilling this and several other compositions, abounding with oily seeds, the operator should be careful not to let the faints mix with the other goods, as they would by that means be rendered nauseous and unsightly; he should therefore be careful towards the latter end of the operation, to catch some of the spirit as it runs from the worm in a glass, and as soon as ever he perceives it the least cloudy, to remove the receiver, and draw the faints by themselves

Of wormwood-water

There are two sorts of wormwood water, distinguished by the epithets of greater and lesser

Receipt for making ten gallons of the lesser composition of wormwood-water

Take the leaves of dried wormwood, five pounds, of the lesser cardamom-seeds, five ounces; draw off ten gallons, or till the faints begin to rise, with a gentle fire. It may be dulcified with sugar, or not, at pleasure. This is a good stomachic and carminative, and on that account, often called for.

Of antiscorbutic water

The scurvy being a disease very common in England, this antiscorbutic water will be of great use.

Receipt for making ten gallons of antiscorbutic water

Take the leaves of water-cresses, garden and sea scurvy-grass, and brookline, of each twenty handfuls; of pine-tops, germander, harehound, and the lesser centaury, of each sixteen handfuls, of the roots of briony and sharp-pointed dock, of each five pounds; of mustard-seed one pound and a half. Digest the whole in ten gallons of proof spirit, and two gallons of water, and draw off by a gentle fire.

This is a good water for the purposes expressed in the title, viz. against scorbutic disorders. It is also good in tremblings, and disorders of the nerves.

Of compound horse-radish water

Take of the fresh roots of horse-radish nine pounds; of the leaves of water-cresses and of garden scurvy-grass, each six pounds; of the outward, or yellow peel of oranges, and lemons, each nine ounces, of winter's bark twelve ounces, of nutmegs three ounces.

Cut,

Cut, bruise and digest the ingredients in ten gallons of proof spirit, and two gallons of water, and draw off ten gallons as before. Or, you may take of the leaves of garden and sea scurvy-grass, fresh gathered in the spring, each seven pounds, brook-lime, water-cresses, and horse-radish-root, of each ten pounds, of winter's bark and nutmegs, each ten ounces, the outer peel of lemons one pound, of arum-root fresh gathered two pounds, proof spirit ten gallons, and two gallons. Bruise and slice the ingredients, digest the whole, and draw off ten gallons as before.

Either of the above receipts will produce an excellent water, against all obstructions of the kidneys and other viscera. It is also of great service in the jaundice, cachexies and dropsies, and in all scorbutic cases, it is equal to any medicine, as it opens the minute passages, promotes transpiration, and clears the skin, and other small glands, which are filled with gross particles, to the detriment of their proper offices.

For making ten gallons of imperial water.

Take of the dried peels of citrons and oranges, of nutmegs, cloves, and cinnamon, each one pound of the roots of cypress, Florentine orrice, calamus aromaticus, each eight ounces, of zedoary, galangal and ginger, of each four ounces; of the tops of lavender and rosemary, each sixteen handfuls, the leaves of white and damask roses, of each twelve handful. Digest the whole two days in ten gallons of proof spirit, and four gallons of damask rose-water, after which draw off ten gallons.

All the ingredients in composition coincide in one intention, and are such as will give their virtues by distillation, circumstances that cannot be said of many other compound waters. It is a very good cephalic, and of great use in all nervous cases. It is also a very pleasant dram, especially if dulcified with fine sugar, and good upon any sudden sickness of the stomach.

Receipt for making ten gallons of compound piony water

Take of the roots of male piony, twelve ounces, of those of wild valerian, nine ounces; and of those of white betony, six ounces, of piony seed, four ounces and a half, of the fresh flowers of lily of the valley, one pound and a half, of those of lavender, Arabian stæchas, and rosemary, each nine ounces; of the tops of betony, marjoram, rue and sage, each six ounces, slice and bruise the ingredients, and digest them four days in ten gallons of proof spirit and two gallons of water; after which draw off ten gallons.

Receipt for two gallons of Eau de Carmes

Take of the fresh leaves of balm, four pounds, of the yellow peel, or rind of lemons, two pounds, of nutmegs and coriander-seeds, each one pound, of cloves, cinnamon, and angelica-root, of each half a pound. Pound the leaves, bruise the other ingredients, and put them with two gallons of fine proof spirit into a large glass alembic, stop the mouth, and place it in a bath-heat to digest two or three days. Then open the mouth of the alembick, and add a gallon of balm-water, and shake the whole well together. After this, place the alembic in Balneum Mariæ, and distil till the ingredients are almost dry, and preserve the water thus obtained in bottles well stopped.

This water has been long famous both at *London* and *Paris*, and carried thence to most parts of *Europe*. It is a very elegant cordial, and of very extraordinary virtues are attributed to it; for it is esteemed very efficacious not only in lowness of spirits, but even in apoplexies; and is greatly commended in cases of the gout in the stomach.

Aqua Mirabilis; or, the wonderful water

Take of cinnamon one pound and a quarter, rind of lemon-peels, ten ounces; cubebs, one ounce and a quarter; leaves of balm, one pound; bruise all these ingredients, and pour on them eleven gallons of clean proof spirit, and one gallon of water, digest the whole twenty-four hours, and distill off ten gallons with a pretty brisk fire; and dulcify it with fine sugar.

Or, take of the lesser cardamoms, cloves, cubebs, galangal, mace, nutmeg, and ginger, of each one pound and three quarters; of the yellow part of citron-peel and cinnamon, of each three pounds and a half; of the leaves of balm one pound; bruise these ingredients, and pour on them eleven gallons of spirit, and one gallon of water; digest, and draw off, &c. as before.

This cordial has been long celebrated as a noble stomachic, and therefore greatly called for.

Receipt for ten gallons of pepper-mint water

Take of dry pepper-mint leaves, fourteen pounds; proof spirit, ten gallons and a half; water one gallon, draw of ten gallons by a gentle fire. You may either dulcify it or not.

Pepper-mint water is a noble stomachic, good against vomiting, nauseas, cholic, and other griping pains in the bowels, in all which intentions it greatly exceeds the common spearmint-water.

Receipt for ten gallons of single Angelica-water

Take of the roots and seed of Angelica, cut and bruised, of each one pound and a half; proof spirit, eleven gallons; draw off ten gallons, or till the faints begin to rise, with a gentle fire, and dulcify it, if required, with lump sugar.

This angelica-water is a good carminative, and therefore good against all kinds of flatulent cholics, and gripings of the bowels.

It may not be amiss to observe here, that in distilling this and several other compositions, abounding only with oily seeds, the operator should be careful not to let the faints mix with the other goods, as they would by that means be rendered nauseous and unsightly; he should therefore be careful towards the latter end of the operation, to catch some of the spirits it runs from the worm in a glass, and as soon as ever he perceives it the least cloudy, to remove the receiver, and draw the faints by themselves.

Of vulnerary-water, or Eau d'Arquebusade.

This vulnerary water is greatly esteemed abroad, and if properly tried, there is no doubt of its obtaining the same reputation here.

Receipt for five gallons of vulnerary-water.

Take of the leaves, flowers and roots of comfrey, leaves of mugwort, sage, and bugle, of each eight handfuls; leaves of betony, sanicle, or ox-eye daisy, the greater figwort, plantain, agrimony, vervain, wormwood, and fennel, of each four handfuls; St. John's wort, birth-wort, orpine, Paul's betony, the lesser centory, yarrow, tobacco, mouse-ear, mint, and hyssop, of each two handfuls; cut them, bruise them well in a mortar, and pour on them three gallons of white wine, and two gallons and a half of proof spirit, digest the whole six days with a gentle heat, in a vessel close stopped; after which distil off with a gentle fire, about five gallons, or till it begins to run milky from the worm.

This water is of excellent service in contusions, tumors, attending dislocations, fractures, and mortifications, the part affected being bathed with it. Some also use it to deterge foul ulcers, and incarn wounds; from whence it was called Vulnerary-Water.

Receipt for a gallon of Bergamot-water

Take the outer rind of three bergamots, a gallon of proof spirit, and two quarts of water. Draw off one gallon in Balneum Mariæ, and dulcify with fine sugar.

If you make your bergamot-water from the essence, or essential oil, be very careful that the spirit be entirely freed from its essential oil; therefore if your spirit be not very cleanly rectified, it will be adviseable to use French brandy. One hundred and sixty drops of the essence will be sufficient for a gallon of spirit, and so in proportion for a greater or smaller quantity.

Receipt for a gallon of the cordial water of Montpellier

Take of the yellow rinds of two bergamots, or fifty drops of the essence of that fruit; cloves and mace, of each half an ounce; proof spirit, a gallon, water one quart. digest two days in a close vessel, draw off a gallon, and dulcify with fine sugar.

Receipt for making a gallon of Honey-water

Take of the best honey and coriander-seeds, of each one pound; cloves, one ounce and a half; nutmegs and gum-benjamin, of each an ounce; vanilloes number four. The yellow rind of three large lemons bruise the cloves, nutmegs, coriander-seeds, and Benjamin; cut the vanilloes in pieces, and put all in a glass alembic, with one gallon of clean rectified spirit, and after digesting forty-eight hours, draw off the spirit in Balneum Mariæ. To a gallon of the above spirit, add of damask rose-water and orange-flower water, of each a pound and a half; musk and ambergrease of each five grains. Grind the musk and ambergrease with some of the water in a glass mortar, and afterwards put altogether into a digesting vessel, shaking them well together, and let them circulate three days and three nights in a gentle heat. then let all cool; filter and keep the water in bottles well stopped, for use.

This

This water was first made by that faithful chemist, Mr. GEORGE WILSON, for King *James* II. It is an anti-paralytic, smooths the skin, and gives one of the most agreeable scents imaginable. Forty or sixty drops put into a pint of clean water, are sufficient for washing the hands and face; and the same proportion to punch, or any cordial water, gives a very agreeable flavour.

Receipt for making a gallon of the common Eau sans Pareille.

Take the outer peels of twelve citrons, three quarts of fine proof spirit, and a quart of water. Put all into a glass alembic, and distil to a dryness in Balneum Mariæ; filtre the water, and put it into bottles, well stopped.

This is the common sort, and what is generally sold here under the name of *Eau sans Pareille.*

Receipt for making a gallon of the best sort of Eau sans Pareille.

Take of the essence of cedrat, bergamot, orange, and lemon, of each two drachms; rectified spirit a gallon; water two quarts. Put all into a glass alembic, and distil in Balneum Mariæ, till the faints begin to rise, when the receiver must be immediately removed.

Of Beauty-water; or Eau de Beauté.

This water has its name from its use in washing the face, and giving an agreeable smell. It is drawn from thyme and marjoram, which gives it a very elegant odour.

Receipt for making a gallon of Beauty-water.

Take of the flowery tops of thyme and marjoram, of each one pound; proof spirits five quarts; water one quart. Draw off in Balneum Mariæ, till the faints begin to rise, and keep it close stopped for use.

Of Royal Water

This water has its name, from being considered as the most excellent of all scented waters. It is compounded of the cedrat, nutmegs and mace, from whence the most elegant smell is produced, and no water is at present thought equal to this. There are two sorts of Royal Water, one produced by a single distillation, and the other by a double distillation, and thence called rectified, or double distilled Royal Water.

Receipt for a gallon of Royal Water

Take of mace one ounce, nutmegs half an ounce, essence of cedrat, or bergamot, two drachms. Put these into a glass alembic (after bruising the spices) with five quarts of fine proof spirit, and draw off one gallon in Balneum Mariæ.

Receipt for making a gallon of double distilled Royal Water

Take of mace one ounce; nutmegs half an ounce; bruise them, and put them into an alembic, with six quarts of fine proof spirit, and draw off five quarts with a gentle fire. Then take the spirit drawn off, and put it into a glass alembic, with two drachms of the essence of cedrat, or bergamot, and draw off a gallon in Balneum Mariæ.

Either of these Receipts will produce an elegant water, but the latter greatly exceeds the former.

Receipt for making a gallon of Bouquet's Water

Take of the flowers of white lilies, and Spanish jessamin, of each half a pound, orange-flowers, and those of the jonquil and pink, of each four ounces, damask roses one pound. Let those be fresh gathered, and immediately put into a glass alembic, with a gallon of clean proof spirit, and two quarts of water. Place the alembic in Balneum Mariæ, draw off till the faints begin to rise. You may use spirit of wine, instead proof spirit; but it will be absolutely necessary that it be entirely inodorous; for otherwise your water will fall short of the desired perfection.

Of Cyprus Water.

This water is only a dilute tincture of ambergrease; but as it is used by those who are fond of that perfume, and known by the name of Cyprus-water, or *Eau de Cypre*, I would not omit giving the receipt here.

Receipt for making a gallon of Cyprus Water

Take of the essence of ambergrease half an ounce; put it into a glass alembic, with a gallon of spirit of wine, and two quarts of water. Place the alembick in Balneum Mariæ, and draw off till the faints begin to rise.

Of Vestal Water, or Eau de Vestale.

This is a very agreeable water, and has been long in use in several parts of *Europe*.

Receipt for a gallon of Vestal Water

Take of the seeds of daucus creticus, or candy carrots, two ounces, spirit of wine, a gallon, water, two quarts. Distil in Balneum Mariæ till the faints begin to rise. Then add the spirit drawn over an ounce of the essence of lemons, and four drops of the essence of ambergrease, re-distil in Balneum Mariæ, and keep the water in bottles well stopped for use.

Receipt for making the Essence of Civet

Take of Civet and double refined sugar, of each two drachms; rub them well together in a glass mortar, adding by degrees five ounces of rectified spirit of wine put the whole into a matrass, digest three days in a gentle heat, and pour off the clear essence for use. Tho the essences here used are, properly speaking, chemical preparations, and therefore foreign to the business of the Distiller, yet as they are often added to perfume waters, and easily made, I thought the above receipts would not be unacceptable to the reader.

Rose-water.

The essence, or essential oil of roses is looked upon as one of the most valuable perfumes in the world, but at the same time the most difficult to be procured in any quantity. A small quantity of it is made in Italy, but it has always been thought impossible to procure it here; and, therefore, a method of acquiring this valuable commodity will not, I presume, be disagreeable to the reader.

Take a quantity of damask rose leaves, put them into a proper vessel, with a sufficient quantity of water, adding some mineral acid, as spirit of salt, vitriol, &c. In this menstruum let the roses be digested for fifteen days; after which put the whole into an alembic, and draw off the water with a pretty brisk fire. But, instead of the common receiver, a separating-glass must be placed under the nose of the worm, and a receiver added to the tube of the separating-glass. By this means all the oil or essence will float on the surface of the water in the separating-glass, and may easily be separated from it, when the operation is finished.

Cinnamon-water, one gallon.

Take a pound of the best cinnamon grosly powdered, digest it for twenty-four hours, in two gallons of water; put the whole into an alembic, and draw over one gallon with a pretty brisk fire.

The oil of cinnamon, in which the specific virtue of the drug consists, is very ponderous, and therefore will not come over the helm unless the fire be pretty brisk, especially with a simple water. It will therefore be in vain to attempt distilling simple cinnamon-water by the *Balneum Mariæ*.

Receipt for making three gallons of compound lavender water.

Take of lavender water two gallons, of hungary water one gallon, cinnamon and nutmegs of each three ounces, and of red saunders one ounce, digest the whole three days in a gentle heat, and then filter it for use. Some add saffron, musk, and ambergrease of each half a scruple; but these are now generally omitted.

This compound lavender water has been long celebrated in all nervous cases. In all kinds of palsies, and loss of memory it is of the greatest service, and has been so much remarked for its efficacy in these complaints, as almost universally to obtain the name of *Palsy Drops*.

Citron-water.

The citron is an agreeable fruit resembling a lemon in colour, smell and taste. The inside is white, fleshy and thick, containing but a small quantity of pulp, in proportion to the bigness of the fruit.

Receipt for making ten gallons of citron water.

Take of dry yellow rinds of citron four pounds, clean proof spirit ten gallons and a half, water one gallon, digest the whole twenty-four hours with a gentle heat; draw off ten gallons, with a gentle fire; or, which is much better, in Balneum Mariæ, and dulcify it with fine sugar to your palate. Or,

Take of dry yellow rinds of citrons three pounds, of orange-peel two pounds, nutmegs bruised three quarters of a pound, digest, draw off, and dulcify as before.

This is one of the most pleasant cordials we have, and the addition of the nutmegs, in the second receipt, increases its virtue as a cephalic and stomachic.

Receipt for one quart of ladies water

Take of sugar candy one pound, of Canary wine six ounces, rose water four ounces; boil them into a syrup, and mix with it of heavenly water one quart, of ambergrise and musk of each eighteen grains, of saffron fifteen grains; yellow saunders two drachms. Digest the whole three days in a vessel close stopped, and decant the clear for use.

This is an extraordinary cordial where the perfumes are not offensive. It is too rich to be drank alone, and therefore should be mixed with water, or some other liquid.

Receipt for a gallon of jasmine water

Take of Spanish jasmine-flowers twelve ounces, essence of florentine citron, or bergamot, eight drops; fine proof spirit a gallon, water two quarts. Digest two days in a close vessel, after which draw off one gallon, and dulcify with fine loaf sugar.

This is a most excellent cordial, and deserves to be more known here than it is at present.

Receipt for a gallon of divine water

Take of orange-flowers fresh gathered two pounds; coriander-seeds three ounces; nutmegs half an ounce, bruise the nutmegs and coriander-seeds; and put them, together with the orange-flowers, into an alembic with a gallon of proof spirit and two quarts of water, draw off the liquor with a gentle fire, till the faints begin to rise, and dulcify with fine sugar.

This is a very pleasant cordial, both with regard to its smell and taste, and on that account in great esteem abroad.

Receipt for making ten gallons of French Usquebagh

Take of saffron three ounces, of the essential oil or essence of florentine citron, bergamot, Portugal orange this and lemon, of each a hundred drops, angelica-seed, vanellos and mace, of each one ounce and a half; cloves and coriander-seed of each three quarters of an ounce, bruise the seeds and spices, and put all into an alembic with eleven gallons of proof spirit, and two gallons of water, and draw off with a gentle fire till the faints begin to rise, fastening to the nose of the worm four ounces of saffron in a cloth. When the operation is finished dulcify the goods with fine sugar.

These waters are excellent cephalic cordials, and alexipharmics, and are excelled by nothing in suddenly reviving the spirits when depressed by sickness, &c.

Of ratafia from peaches

The ratafia made from the peach is of the finest and richest flavour of any made from stoned fruits. It is however necessary to gather the peach when thoroughly ripe, but, at the same time not to suffer it to hang too long on the tree. For as, on the one hand, it will not acquire its delicate flavour and smell till thoroughly ripe, so, on the other it will lose both if suffered to hang on the tree, after it has attained to a full maturity ———— Another necessary caution is, to gather them in fine warm weather, and near the middle of the day, because then both the flavour and smell are in the greatest perfection. For this the best flavoured fruits must be chose.

Receipt for making ten gallons of common ratafia

Take of nutmegs eight ounces, bitter almonds ten pounds, Lisbon sugar eight pounds, ambergrise ten grains. Infuse these ingredients three days in ten gallon of clean proof spirit, and filtre thro' a flannel bag for use.

The nutmegs and bitter almonds must be bruised; and the ambergrise rubbed with the Lisbon sugar in a marble mortar, before they are infused in the spirit.

Fennel-

Fennel-water, a gallon

Take one pound of sweet fennel-seeds, and two gallons of water; put them into an alembic, and draw off one gallon with a gentle fire.

Pepper-mint-water

Pepper-mint is a very celebrated stomachic, and on that account greatly used at present, and its simple water often called for.

Pepper-mint-water

Take of the leaves of dried pepper-mint, one pound and a half, water two gallons and a half; put all into an alembic, and draw off one gallon, with a gentle fire.

The water obtained from pepper-mint by distillation in Balneum Mariæ, is more fragrant and more fully impregnated with the virtues of the plant than that drawn by the alembic. The same may be said with regard to that extracted by the cold still; when the cold still is used the plant must be green, and if possible committed to the still with the morning dew upon it.

Spear-mint-water.

Spear-mint is also like pepper-mint a great stomachic, and therefore constantly used.

Spear-mint-water, one gallon

Take of the leaves of dried spear-mint one pound and a half; water two gallons and a half, draw off by a gentle fire one gallon.

This water, like that drawn from peppermint, will be more fragrant if distilled in Balneum Mariæ, or the cold still; but if the latter be used, the same caution must be observed of distilling the plant green.

Receipt

Receipt for a gallon of cedrat water with the essence of the fruit

Take of the finest loaf sugar reduced to powder a quarter of a pound, put it into a glass mortar, with one hundred and twenty drops of the essence of cedrat, rub them together with a glass pestle, put them into a glass alembic with a gallon of fine proof spirits and a quart of water. Place the alembic in Balneum Mariæ, and draw off one gallon, or till the faints being to rise, and dulcify with fine sugar.

You must be very careful that the spirit be entirely freed from its essential oil, and therefore if your spirit be not very cleanly rectified, it will be adviseable to use French brandy, lest the fine flavour so highly esteemed in this cordial be destroyed by the spirit.

Almond butter.

Take a quart of cream, put in some mace whole, and a quartered nutmeg, yolks of eight eggs well beaten, and three quarters of a pound of almonds well blanched, and beaten extremely small, with a little rosewater and sugar, put all these together, set them on the fire, and stir them till they begin to boil; then take it off, and you will find it a little crack'd, so lay a strainer in a colander, and pour it into it, and let it drain a day or two, till you see it is firm like butter; then run it through a colander, then it will be like little comfits, and so serve it up.

Clouted cream

Take a gill of new milk, and set it on the fire, and take six spoonfuls of rosewater, four or five pieces of large mace, put the mace on a thread; when it boils, put to them the yolks of two eggs very well beaten; stir these very well together, then take a quart of very good cream, put it to the rest, and stir it together, but let it not boil after the cream is in. Pour it out of the pan you boil it in, and let it stand all night; the next day take the top of it, and serve it up.

Citron

Citron cream

Take a quart of cream, and boil it with three penny worth of good clear isinglass, which must be tied up in a piece of thin taffaty; put in a blade or two of mace strongly boiled in your cream and isinglass, till the cream be pretty thick; sweeten it to your taste, with perfumed hard sugar, when it is taken off the fire, put in a little rosewater to your taste, then take a piece of your green freshest citron, and cut it in little bits, the breadth of point-dales, and about half as long, and the cream being first put into dishes, when it is half cold, put in your citron, so as it may but sink from the top, that it may not be seen, and may lie before it be at the bottom; if you wash your citron before in rosewater, it will make the colour better and fresher, so let it stand till the next day, where it may get no water, and where it may not be shaken

Conserve of roses boiled

Take red roses, take off the whites at the bottom or elsewhere, take three times the weight of them in sugar, put to a pint of roses a pint of water, skim it well, shred your roses a little before you put them into water, cover them, and boil the leaves tender in the water, and when they are tender, put in your sugar, keep them stirring, lest they burn when they are tender, and the syrup consumed. Put them up, and so keep them for use

To make cordial poppy water

Take two gallons of very good brandy, and a peck of poppies, and put them together in a wide-mouth'd glass, and let them stand forty-eight hours, and then strain the poppies out; take a pound of raisins of the sun, stone them, and an ounce of coriander-seeds, and an ounce of sweet fennel seeds, and an ounce of liquorice sliced, bruise them all together, and put them into

to the brandy, with a pound of good powdered sugar, and let them stand four or eight weeks, shaking it every day, and then strain it off, and bottle it close up for use.

Of the simple waters commonly in Use.

Simple waters are not so much used at present as they formerly were, and perhaps one reason for their being neglected, is the bad methods used in distilling them; the process is carried on in the same manner with every herb; though some should be gently dried, and others distilled green, some should be drawn with the cold, and others with the hot still.

The general rule that should be observed with regard to the hot still is, that all herbs should have twice their weight of water added to them in the still, and not above a fourth, or a sixth part of it drawn off again; for simple waters have their faints, if drawn too low, as well as those that are spirituous.

Some plants, particularly balm, require to have the water drawn from them cohobated, or poured several times on a fresh parcel of the herb, in order to give it a proper degree of strength or richness. Others, on the contrary, abound too much with an essential oil, that floats on the distilled water; in this case all the oil should be carefully taken off. Lastly, those that contain a more fixed oil, should be imperfectly fermented, before they are distilled; of this kind are carduus, camomile, &c.

The simple waters now commonly made, are orange-flower-water, rose-water, cinnamon-water, fennel-water, pepper-mint-water, spear-mint-water, balm-water, pennyroyal-water, Jamaica pepper-water, castor-water, simple-water of orange-peel, and of dill-seed.

Of Faints, and the Uses they may be applied to.

In many of the preceding receipts, I have ordered the receiver to be removed as soon as the faints begin

to

to rise; because otherwise the goods would contract a disagreeable taste and smell. It is not however to be understood that these faints are to be thrown away, nor the working of the still immediately stopped, for they are far from being of no value, notwithstanding they would be of great disadvantage, if suffered to run among the more spirituous parts of the goods before drawn off. As soon therefore as you find the clear colour of the goods begins to change of a bluish or whitish colour, remove the receiver, place another under the nose of the worm, and continue the distillation as long as the liquor running from the worm is spirituous, which may be known by pouring a little of it on the still-head, and applying a lighted candle to to it, for if it is spirituous it will burn, but otherwise not. When the faints will no longer burn on the still-head, put out the fire, and pour the faints in a cask for that purpose; and, when from repeated distillations, you have procured a sufficient quantity of these faints, let the still be charged with them almost to the top. Then throw into the still three or four pounds of salt, and draw off as you would any other charge, as long as the spirit extracted is of a sufficient strength, after which the receiver is to be removed, and the faints saved by themselves as before.

The spirits thus extracted from the faints will serve in several compositions as well as fresh; but they are generally used in Anniseed-water, because the predominant taste of the Anniseeds, will entirely cover that they had before acquired from other ingredients.

Directions for making a luting for stills

By the term luting an alembic, we mean, the closing the joints through which the spirits might transpire.

Lute is a composition of common ashes, well sifted, and soaked in water; clay, and a kind of paste made of meal or starch are also used for this purpose, which as before observed, is to close all the joints, &c. in order to confine the spirits from transpiring.

Direction

Directions for the use of the cold still

As the method of performing the operation by the cold still, is the very same, whatever plant or flower is used, the following instance of procuring a water from rosemary, will be abundantly sufficient to instruct the young practitioner in the manner of conducting the process in all cases whatever

Take rosemary, fresh gathered, in its perfection, with the morning due upon it, and lay it lightly and unbruised upon the plate, or bottom of the still Cover the plate with its conical head, and apply a glass receiver to the nose of it Make a small fire of charcoal under the plate, continuing it as long as any liquor comes over into the receiver When nothing more comes over, take off the still head, and remove the plant, putting fresh in its stead, and proceed as before, continue to repeat the operation succeffively, till a sufficient quantity of water is procured Let this distilled water be kept at rest, in clean bottles, close stopped for some days in a cold place; by this mean it will become limpid, and powerfully impregnated with the taste and smell of the plant

How to make Blackberry Wine.

Take your berries when full ripe, put them into a large vessel of wood or stone, with a spicket in it, and pour upon them as much boiling water as will just appear on the top of them, as soon as you can endure your hand in them bruise them very well, till all the berries be broke; then let them stand close covered till the berries be well wrought up to the top, which usually is three or four days, then draw off the clear juice into another vessel, and add to every ten quarts of this liquor one pound of sugar, stir it well in, and let it stand to work in another vessel like the first, a week or ten days, then draw it off at the spicket through a jelly-bag, into a large vessel, take four ounces of isinglass, lay it in steep twelve hours in a pint of white wine; the next morning boil it till it be

all

all diſſolved, upon a ſlow fire, then take a gallon of your blackberry juice, put in the diſſolved iſinglaſs, give it a boil together, and put it in hot

How to make Orange Wafers

Take the beſt oranges, and boil them in three or four waters, till they be tender; then take out the kernels and the juice, and beat them to pulp, in a clean marble mortar, and rub them through a hair ſieve; to a pound of this pulp take a pound and a half of double-refined ſugar, beaten and ſearſed; take half of your ſugar, and put it into your oranges, and boil it till it rope, then take it from the fire, and when it is cold, make it up in paſte with the other half of your ſugar, make but little at a time, for it will dry too faſt, then with a little rolling-pin roll them out as thin as tiffany upon papers, cut them round with a little drinking-glaſs, and let them dry, and they will look very clear

How to make Cyder.

After all your apples are bruiſed, take half of your quantity and ſqueeze them, and the juice or preſs from them pour upon the others half bruiſed, but not ſqueezed, in a tub for the purpoſe, having a tap at the bottom, let the juice remain upon the apples three or four days, then pull out your tap, and let your juice run into ſome other veſſel ſet under the tap to receive it; and if it run thick, as at the firſt it will pour it upon the apples again, till you ſee it run clear; and as you have a quantity, put it into your veſſel but do not force the cyder, but let it drop as long as it will of its own accord Having done this, after you perceive that the ſides begin to work, take a quantity of iſinglaſs, an ounce will ſerve for forty gallons; infuſe this into ſome of the cyder till it be diſſolved; put to an ounce of iſinglaſs a quart of cyder; and when it is ſo diſſolved, pour it into the veſſel, and ſtop it cloſe for two days, or ſomething more, then draw off the cyder into another veſſel this do ſo often till you perceive your cyder to be free from

from all manner of sediment, that may make it ferment and fret itself After Christmas you may boil it, you may, by pouring water on the apples, and pressing them, make a pretty small cyder; if it be thick and muddy, by using isinglass, you may make it as clear as the rest, you must dissolve the isinglass over the fire, till it be jelly

How to make fine Almond Cakes.

Take a pound of Jordan almonds, blanch them, beat them very fine with a little orange-flower water, to keep them from oiling, then take a pound and a quarter of fine sugar, boil it to a high candy, then put in your almonds; then take two fresh lemons, grate off the rind very thin, and put as much juice as to make it of a quick taste, then put it into your glasses, and set it into your stove, stirring them often that they do not candy so, when it is a little dry, put it into little cakes upon sheets of glass to dry.

How to make yellow varnish

Take a quart of spirit of wine, and put to it eight ounces of seed-cake, shake it half an hour; next day it will be fit for use, but strain it first, take lamp-black, and put in your varnish about the thickness of a pancake, mix it well, but stir it not too fast; then do it eight times over, and let it stand till the next day; then take some burn'd ivory, and oil of turpentine as fine as butter, then mix it with some of your varnish, till you have varnished it fit for polishing, then polish it with Tripola in fine flour, then lay it on the wood smooth, with one of the brushes; then let it dry, and do it so eight times at the least, when it is very dry lay on your varnish that is mixed, and when it is dry, polish it with a wet cloth dipped in Tripola, and rub it as hard as you would do platters

How to make a pretty varnish to colour little baskets, bowls, or any board where nothing hot is set on

Take either red, black or white wax, which colour you want to make; to every two ounces of sealing-wax one ounce of spirit of wine, pound the wax fine, then sift it through a fine lawn sieve, till you have

made

made it extremely fine, put it into a large phial with the spirit of wine, shake it, let it stand within the air of the fire forty-eight hours, shaking it often, then with a little brush rub your baskets all over with it, let it dry, and do it over a second time, and it makes them look very pretty

How to clean gold or silver lace

Take alabaster finely beaten and searsed, and put it into an earthen pipkin, and set it upon a chafing-dish of coals, and let it boil for some time, stirring it often with a stick first; when it begins to boil, it will be very heavy; when it is enough, you will find it in the stirring very light, then take it off the fire, lay your lace upon a piece of flannel, and strew your powder upon it; knock it well in with a hard cloth brush, when you think it is enough, brush the powder out with a clean brush

How to make sweet Powder for Cloaths

Take orris roots, two pound and a half, of lignum rodicum, six ounces of scraped cypress roots, three ounces, of damask roses, carefully dried, a pound and a half of Benjamin, four ounces and a half of storax, two ounces and a half of sweet marjoram, three ounces of labdanum, one ounce and a drachm of calamus aromaticus, and one drachm of musk cods, six drachms of lavender and flowers, and melilot flowers, if you please

To clean white sattins, flowered silks, with gold and silver in them

Take stale bread crumbled very fine, mixed with powder-blue, rub it very well over the silk and sattin, then shake it well, and with clean soft cloths dust it well. If any gold or silver flowers, afterwards take a piece of crimson in grain velvet and rub the flowers with it

To keep arms, Iron or steel from rusting

Take the filings of lead, or dust of lead, finely beaten in an iron mortar, putting to it oil of spike, which will make the iron smell well, and if you oil your arms, or any thing that is made of iron or steel, you may keep them in moist airs from rusting

To make Spanish Fritters.

Take the inside of a roll, and slice it in three; then soak it in milk, then pass it through a batter of eggs, fry them in butter, when almost done, repass them in another batter; then let them fry till they are done, draw them off the butter, and lay them in a dish, over every pair of fritters you must throw cinnamon, small coloured sugar plumbs, and clarified sugar.

How to make little French Biscuits

Take nine new-layed eggs, take the yolks of two out, and take out the tredles, beat them a quarter of an hour, and put in a pound of searsed sugar, and beat them together three quarters of an hour, then put in three quarters of a pound of flour, very fine and well dried. When it is cold, mix all well together, and beat them about half a quarter of an hour at last. If you please put in a little orange-flower water, and a little grated lemon-peel, then drop them about the bigness of half-a-crown, (but rather long than round) upon doubled paper a little buttered, sierce some sugar on them, and bake them in an oven, after manchets.

The Stag's Heart Water.

Take balm four handfuls, sweet marjoram one handful, rosemary flowers, clove-gilliflowers dried, red rose buds, borrage flowers, of each an ounce; marygold flowers, half an ounce, lemon-peel two ounces, mace and cardimum, of each thirty grains; of cinnamon sixty grains, of yellow and white sanders, of each a quarter of an ounce, shavings of hart's-horn an ounce, take nine oranges, and put in the peel; then cut them in small pieces, pour upon these two quarts of the best Rhenish, or the best white wine; let it infuse three or four days, being very close stopped in a cellar or cool place. If it infuse nine or ten days, it is the better.

To make Slip-Coat Cheese

Take six quarts of new milk hot from the cow, the froathings, and put to it two spoonfuls of rennet, and when

when it is hard coming, lay it into the fat with a spoon, not breaking it at all; then press it with a four pound weight, turning it with a dry cloth once an hour, and every day shifting it on fresh grass. It will be ready to cut, if the weather be hot, in fourteen days.

A powder for the heartburn.

Take white chalk six ounces, eyes and claws of crabs, of each an ounce, oil of nutmeg six drops, make them into a fine powder. About a drachm of this in a glass of cold water, is an infallible cure for the heartburn.

A fine lip salve.

Take two ounces of virgin's-wax, two ounces of hog's-lard, half an ounce of spermaceti, one ounce of oil of sweet-almonds, two drams of balsam of Peru, two drams of alkenet root cut small, six new raisins shred small, a little fine sugar, simmer them all together a little while; then strain it off into little pots. It is the finest lip salve in the world.

To make Carolina snow balls.

Take half a pound of rice, wash it clean, divide it into six parts; take six apples, pare them and scoop out the core, in which place put a little lemon-peel shred very fine, then have ready some thin cloaths to tie the balls in; put the rice in the cloth, and lay the apple on it, tie them up close; put them into cold water, and when the water boils, they will take an hour and a quarter boiling; be very careful how you turn them into the dish, that you don't break the rice, and they will look as white as snow, and make a very pretty dish ——— The sauce is, to this quantity, a quarter of a pound of fresh butter, melted thick, a wine-glass of white wine, a little nutmeg and beaten cinnamon, made very sweet with sugar; boil all up together, and pour it into a bason, and send to table.

How to make almond milk for a wash.

Take five ounces of bitter almonds, blanch them and beat them in a marble mortar very fine. You must put in a spoonful of sack, when you beat them; then take the whites of three new-layed eggs, three pints of spring-water, and one pint of sack. Mix there all very well, then strain it through a fine cloth, and put

... to a bottle, and keep it for use. You may put in ... or powder of pearl when you make use of it.

To make orange loaves

Take your oranges, and cut a round hole in the top, ... all the meat, and as much of the white as you can without breaking the skin; then boil them in water till tender, shifting the water till 'tis not bitter; then take them up and wipe them dry, then take a pound of fine sugar, a quart of water, or in proportion to the oranges, boil it, and take off the scum as it ...eth, then put in your oranges, and let them boil a little and let them lie a day or two in the syrup, then take the yolks of two eggs, a quarter of a pint of cream, (or more) beat them well together, then grate in two Naples biscuits, (or white bread) a quarter of a pound of butter, and four spoonfuls of sack, mix it all together till your butter is melted; then fill the oranges with it, and bake them in a slow oven as long as you would a custard; then stick in some cut citron, and fill them up with sack, butter, and sugar grated over.

To candy Angelica

Take it in April, boil it in water till it be tender; then take it up and drain it from the water very well, then scrape the outside of it, and dry it in a clean cloth, and lay it in the syrup, and let it lie in three or four days, and cover it close, the syrup must be strong of sugar, and keep it hot a good while, and let it not boil; after it is heated a good while, lay it upon a pye-plate, and so let it dry, keep it near the fire, lest it dissolve.

Sack cream like butter

Take a quart of cream, boil it with mace, put to it six egg-yolks well beaten, so let it boil up; then take it off the fire, and put in a little sack, and turn it, then put it in a cloth, and let the whey run from it; then take it out of the cloth, and season it with rose-water and sugar, being very well broken with a spoon; serve it up in the dish, and pink it as you would do a dish of butter, so send it in with cream and sugar.

To join china

Take oyster-shell powder, and the white of an egg, beat it as fine as possible; then mix the powder and the white of an egg, as thick as white paint, then take your china, and lay it on pretty thick, and then hold it close with your hands, before a good fire, till the china is hot, and it will be fastened in two minutes, then pour boiling water into it directly, then wipe it dry, and with a penknife scrape it clean on both sides, and it will appear only as a crack, you must be very quick in doing it; otherwise the remainder that is left to join the rest of the china, will grow hard and be of no use, if either the heat of the fire or wind comes near it.

How to make the oystershell-powder

Take a large deep shell, put it in the middle of a very good clear fire, and burn it, till it is red hot, then carefully take it out with a pair of tongs, scrape all the black away, and then pound it in a mortar, till it is as fine as a powder, then sift it through a fine linen cloth, till you have made it as fine as possibly you can.

To join glass

Take alabaster, pound it, and rub it in a mortar with the pestle, then sift it through a fine linen cloth, and mix it with the white of an egg, as you do for the china, join it, and hold it at a proper distance from the fire, so as not to break the glass, then with a knife scrape off what sticks without side.

N B Gum-arabic steeped in boiling water, made to a proper thickness, will do the same thing.

THE
New ART of Brewing
AND
Improving MALT LIQUORS
To the greatest Advantage.

CONTAINING

[The] New Improvement of [the] Barley Corn, for ma[k]ing the best, and palest [M]alt.
[The] best Methods of brew[in]g all Sorts of fine Ale, [s]trong Beer, and Table [B]eer, in several Parts of [E]ngland and Wales.
[An] Account of Hops, and of [a] new discovered Herb [g]rowing wild, which for [its] agreeable bitter, and wholesome qualities, is often preferred to the Hop.
Curious Methods of drying Malt and Hops in the greatest Perfection.
How to prevent the Damage done by the Wevil Insect, to Malt, Wheat, &c.
To fine, relish, strengthen and preserve Ale or strong Beer, Wine or Cyder, and to recover them if turned, &c. &c. &c.

[Wit]h many other curious and very useful Matters rela[t]ing to the BREWERY, never before published.

[And] absolutely necessary for all who would brew their own MALT DRINK in the highest Perfection.

By WILLIAM ELLIS,
Late of London, Brewer.

DUBLIN.

[Prin]ted by JOHN EXSHAW, at the BIBLE in Dame-street, opposite Castle-lane.
MDCCLXI

THE
New Art of Brewing
AND
Improving Malt Liquors

To the greatest Advantage

How to have Barley of a white Colour

IF the crop is let to stand till the ears are full bent, and the crop full ripe, the kernels will be reddish, and thick-skinned therefore, when the ear and kernel looks a little bluish and a little spotted, and the ear out just bent, then mow it, and it will thus contribute much to the kernels whiteness

How to try Barley, whether it will make good Malt or not

It was the practice of an eminent malster, when he doubted the goodness of his barley, to---put an handful in water, enough to cover it, and let it soak five tides, twelve hours being a tide, and at the end take it out, and let it lay near the fire twenty-four hours;

hours;—then if it begins to sprout, which it will do in that time if at all, it is good,—otherwise, that which does not sprout, will not answer for malt

Brewing Strong Beer or Ale with Bruised Malt

This is to be done by a new method of brewing with whole malt kernels only bruised in a little hand mill, made with wood and iron, which being turned by a handle, the two small wooden rollers plated with iron receive the malt out of a wooden hopper, and gradually bruise and discharge the kernels in its working. Thus they are prepared for imbibing the scalding water, which they will much sooner do than ground malt; because, by such bruising, the malt kernels are directly brought into spungy bodies, provided the malt is leisurely dried mellow. For if the kernels are scorched into a hardness, they will not rightly answer this purpose; but if in right order, they will presently and regularly discharge all the virtue of the malt in making only a strong ale or beer. For this——the water must be first put into the mash tub, as soon as it just begins to boil; and when in, you must directly put your malt leisurely on it, while another keeps stirring it to mix it well with the water. If you brew four bushels and a half of such malt, reserve the half bushel to cap and cover the mashed four, for lying undisturbed two hours. At the end of which time, lade over bowls full of scalding, or near boiling water now and then, and continue so doing till you thus draw off what quantity of strong wort you think fit, letting the wort run all the while, by a very small stream, on fresh hops, confined in a fine net or coarse canvas bag. At last, put wort and hops into your copper, where after they have been boiled thirty minutes, take out the hops, but boil your wort till it breaks into large particles as big in appearance as grain of corn, which it will the sooner do, if at it's first boiling you put into it a large spoonful of common salt dissolved in a pint of water, and the whole furiously boiled. Thus you may draw off a barrel or thirty two gallons of strong ale or keeping beer, from only this quantity of malt, and have it in a fine potent healthy condition, more free from that earthy phlegmatick quality attending the fediment of ground malt, becaufe the bruifed malt kernels become fo many ftrainers to the wort, and caufe it to come off tranfparently fine, and much the ftronger, as their virtue is altogether expended in making only a ftrong ale or ftrong beer. for thus there is no goodnefs left in the malt or grains for fmall beer

N B If you put an ounce of true falt of tartar into about an hogfhead of the hot water, before you mafh the bruifed malt, it will extract the virtue of the malt the fooner and better, and will help to fine and preferve the liquor, and is very wholefome

A new method that gets more and more into Practice for brewing a Family Small-Beer from freſh Malt ground

This is practifed by boiling frefh hops in a roomy fine net, or in a large canvas bag, half an hour, when they are to be taken out of the copper, and the boiled water put in the mafh tub, there to remain till the fiery vapour is a little abated Then put your malt leifurely into it, leaving only a little to cap and cover the mafh. let all reft undifturbed for two hours or more, then draw off the wort. If you think fit, you may mafh a fecond time with more boiling hot water; or do it by lading bowls full of it, till all the goodnefs of the malt is wafhed out, in making an entire family fmall beer When the wort is cooled enough, put about two or three quarts of it in an earthen pan, with yeaft, and when this has worked enough, add it to the reft of the wort, before it is cold, and you will have, if the malt was in right order, a pleafant wholefome fmall table beer

How to brew a Strong Ale or beer without boiling Wort or Hops

Let your water be juft ready to boil, then put as much into your mafh tub as will but thoroughly wet the malt here let it remain undisturbed about a quarter of an hour, the better for disposing the malt to give out its virtue or sweetness to the hot water, which is at the end of that time to be put over it boiling hot, to the quantity as much as you would use for your first wort; mash it well, and let it remain undisturbed under cover, two hours; then put what quantity of hops you think fit into your receiver, and let your wort run on them. Here, after your hops have been infused an hour and half in your wort, strain it off to your coolers. Next, you are to mash the malt with more boiling water for making a second wort, and then let it lie undisturbed only one hour, at the end of which run it off on more fresh hops as they lie loose in your receiver, as your first wort did; then put your first and second worts, with all their hops, into your copper, where they are to lie and infuse till your wort is near boiling, but does not boil; then strain it into your coolers, and your brewing thus a strong ale or beer is finished till it is worked and fermented.

If you will make a small beer after this strong, you may put over cold water on the grains and mash them, which is to remain only one hour, and draw it off up on fresh hops; and if you think fit, you may manage this in the same manner you did the strong drink, by only heating the wort and hops in the copper, or boil it, as in the common way.

This water not boiled does not lose it spirits, for boiling opens its body, and lets the spirits on the wing, leaving it cold and harsh, and of a hard nature, therefore it will not prepare any food or drink so natural, nor to that advantage, as that water which hath not boiled. To prove this, boil a good quantity of river water, and put it into a clean vessel, and let it stand a while, and then take a like quantity of unboiled raw water, and put it into another vessel, and let it stand the same time, and you will find the boiled water to sink, and never to be sweet again. But your other water, which remains intire, and not touched with the fire, will also stink or rather ferment, and then will be sweet and good as before for any use, especially that
of

of the non-such river Thames——The reason therefore is this; the fire doth force out and evaporate the essential spirit and preserving virtue, which renders it of a phlegmatick dead gross nature and taste; but that is only raw which is not digested, and is not the drink I recommend here, for this has passed through all the digestions and fermentations it ought to do; but few will believe this, because custom too often prevails over reason

N. B. The quantity of hops for unboiled strong wort should be seven pounds to nine bushels of malt for a hogshead of strong beer; but for ale, only two or three is enough

The best Method of Brewing Ale or strong Beer, by boiling Water, Wort, and Hops.

I will suppose, that I am to brew half a hogshead, or twenty-seven gallons of strong keeping beer, from four bushels and half of malt, not ground too small, and also as much small beer after the strong. In the first place, if I am to brew brown malt, I would endeavour to have that which has been dried on the kiln at least six hours——If an amber malt, ten——If a pale, twenty hours at least. I would also use soft pond, or river water for the brown malt; but for amber or pale, hard water from the spring; but whether it be of the hard or soft sort, as soon as it is put into the copper, I would have it strewed over with a handful or two of ground malt, or bran, or meal. If the water is hard, it will soften it, if soft, it will soften it more; then when it has just boiled, put it in your mash tub, and let it stand till you can see your face in it, then begin to put your four bushels of malt very leisurely into it, stir it and mash it well, to prevent clotting and lying in some parts dry; mash for a quarter of an hour, and then spread the remaining half bushel of dry malt over the whole to keep in the spirit of the rest, to lie thus two hours or more. then let your cock run a small stream, and return it until the wort comes off fine into your receiver on fresh hops, and as it thus runs off, lade over more boiling water very leisurely from time to time, for the gradual washing out the virtue of the malt. And for carrying on this brewing the safer, the two coppers or kettles hereafter mentioned, should be furnished with boiling water; that when one is expended on the malt, and the first wort put into the copper with hops in a net or bag; I say, while the first wort and hops are boiling, the water in the other copper or kettle may be continued lading over the malt, as the first was for making a second strong wort,—or the boiling wort may be put on the malt all at once and mashed, for lying only one hour undisturbed. Then the second wort is likewise to run into the receiver on fresh hops. And when the first wort has been boiled half an hour, take out the bag of hops, but boil the wort on till it breaks, at which crisis of time, the wort is to be put into coolers; then boil your second wort and hops as the first was, and empty it into your coolers; so have you a strong drink brewed and for small, make use of cold water to mash with, and after an hour's lying draw off, and boil it with fresh hops one hour or more——To work and ferment this, the former directions will serve.

For thus making use of two coppers or kettles in brewing, all authors besides myself have omitted giving an account of their excellent service; for although four or five bushels of malt are brewed, the second copper or kettle is absolutely necessary towards preserving the malt and wort in a right sweetness; else an acute brewer, much more an ignorant one, is very liable to have his hot liquor or wort sour on his grains, and that would be an irretrievable damage, as it cannot by any means be recovered. This, therefore is regarded by the workman, as one of the chief points of his skill to prevent.

How to brew a Double Ale or Strong Beer, called
Norfolk Nog

Boil your water as long as any scum will arise, which scum you must cast away. Then set your water to cool

cool till it is of a right heat; which, to be exactly informed of, it is when the steam or reek has left the hot water, and you can easily see your face in it. As soon as your water is ready, you must put the quantity sufficient to make a hogshead of ale, or rather a barrel containing thirty-two gallons, upon five bushels of malt, which before you let run must stand an hour and half. When drawn off, you may directly put it into another tub, in which three bushels of malt and two of the best wheat bran mixt together were first put. Stir it well, let it stand an hour longer after you have strewed some bran or dry malt over its surface. Then cover it close with cloths to prevent the heat from evaporating, else it may be too cold to extract the virtue of the malt. When you draw it off, put it into the copper with a quart of dry malt more; and boil the whole as long as any white froth ariseth on it, which will be in three quarters of an hour; though it won't hurt it, but rather add to its strength and goodness, were it to boil longer in the copper. One good handful of hops is enough for a hogshead, which should be put into your copper.

If you chuse to have fine beer made without hops, a pound of good ginger well beaten or ground with a mill, and boiled along with the beer, will render it much more wholesome, and less liable to spoil in keeping. As soon as your beer has boiled as long as you think fit, draw it off, and set it by to cool in open shallow tubs made on purpose, then put a pint of yeast to a quart of the beer lukewarm, or less than blood-warm, and by degrees mix and work the whole brewing, observing that it be not too hot when the yeast is put in, the consequence of which will be, the drink will be affected with a disagreeable taste. On the other hand, if it be too cold, it will not work at all, and you will be obliged in frosty and cold weather to warm it over the fire before the yeast will have the desired heat ———— If you intend your beer for keeping, you may turn it within six hours after it has acquired a head. But if you design it for speedy drinking, let it stand full twelve hours.

As the virtue of the eight bushels of malt can't be wholly extracted by one hogshead of water, you may take the five bushels of malt and the three bushels that were mixed with two of bran, and putting them together mash them over again, and set aside the first running for ale, and the second for small beer.

The ingenious Contrivance of a petty Country Publican, for brewing a stronger Ale or Beer than other, from the same Quantity of Malt.

He provided himself with two large kettles, and commonly brewed only five bushels of malt at a time and when he had thus brewed his strong and small drink from the same, he barrelled up his strong, but reserved his small beer wort unfermented, to be made use of as the first hot water to be put over the new five bushels of ground malt, which he directly brewed after he had brewed his first And when he had brewed this last, he worked his strong and small beer with yeast as usual; and thus made only one barrel of small beer from his two brewings, and a much better and stronger ale.

How an Innkeeper brewed his strong or Double Beer, which he sold for Sixpence per Quart.

This Person having a copper that boiled off a hogshead at a time; in *March* and *October* he commonly brewed his strong stout sixpenny beer, a butt containing two hogsheads at a time, thus about three o'clock in the afternoon he began to brew his first quantity of malt, viz twelve bushels, and when his water or liquor had just broke into a boil, he put it into his mash tun, here to lie till the fiery vapour is spent He then put into it by degrees his first twelve bushels of ground malt, and after mashing it, let it he covered an hour and a half, when he drew off his first wort, and put it into his copper with six pounds of hops and as the second copper of hot water was heating while the first mash lay under cover, he put it over the malt, mashed it, and let it lie covered an hour and a half, and boiled his first wort till it broke into large particles, which it did in about half an hour's time with a fierce furze fire And when his second wort was drawn off, he immediately put cold water over the grains, mashed the and let them stand an hour and half. Now his first wort being put into coolers, he reserved his second wort unboiled for an after-management, and took his small beer wort into his copper to boil instead of a first hot water for brewing his second twelve bushels of malt, which was done directly after the first twelve bushels were brewed off as aforesaid; and when this first small beer wort was broke into a boil he put it into his mash tun, and when a little cooled he put in his malt and mashed it for letting it lie under cover an hour and half; then mashed the malt a second time with a copper of hot water for making a second wort, after the first wort of the second twelve bushels is boiled off. This second wort goes into the copper with the reserved second wort of the first twelve bushels, both quantities making a hogshead, which being boiled with all the twelve pounds of the first used hops, it made a hogshead of common ale. At last he mashed up with cold water and drawing off about thirty gallons, he boiled it with some of the refuse hops for small beer which he sold to poor people——Thus he made of twenty four bushels of malt one butt of sixpenny beer, and one hogshead of groat ale, with but little small beer; somewhat after the manner they brew their Norfold Nog, which is the best butt beer, and the worst of common ale, because the last is brewed with only the dregs of the malt and hops.

Of Hops, and an Account of a new invented Malt and Hop Kiln, and of Herbs that supply the Use of Hops.

At the beginning of *September*, or somewhat sooner hops become brownish, and ready for gathering. In this case a sufficient number of hands should not be wanting, for the quicker the hops are gathered, the sooner they will be out of the danger of being too ripe, and of foul weather——If the plantation be a large one, there must be huts or sheds erected to secure the hops from rain, and for lodging the gatherers.

ers. Hops must not be gathered in the dew nor rain, and as they are picked off the poles, that are brought and laid across the binn or frame, they are to be cleared from all leaves and other trumpery; and to prevent their sweating, they should be soon tied up in cloths, or otherwise, and carried to the kiln. The common malt kiln is made use of in some places, by burning charcoal under the hops that lye on an hair cloth, but the following far exceeds it.

Some have recommended several sorts of herbs for supplying the use of hops, and say that for many constitutions they are much better; for that it is custom more than the real virtues of the hop that renders them in general use and esteem. It is true that hops are a most serviceable vegetable in brewing, if rightly managed, and would be better if they could be dryed only by the sun; but as this cannot be conveniently done, a late invention of doing it is, I think, the nearest of any way, which is by drying hops on the cockle oast kiln, as I have seen near Canterbury that performs their drying entirely by hot air, free of any pernicious vapour from the fire, though dryed from the rankest fewel. Malt is also dryed from the same kiln in the greatest perfection of sweetness, for here it is dryed very leisurely, especially the pale sort, because it cannot be here scorched, discoloured or tang'd by smoke. Therefore I am sure that many gentlemen would have their malt dryed on such a kiln, if they were sensible of the great advantage attending its uses. It is true that the common malster thinks this kiln rather too slow a drying for his profit; but if they would undertake it, many would be glad to give an advanced price for it, for at present there is thought to be hardly one quarter of malt in fifty that is rightly made throughout the kingdom ——Herbs said to supply hops are the pennyroyal, balm, tansy, wormwood, broom, carduus, centaury, betony, dandelion, bay leaves, buckbean, horehound, &c but no author has taken notice of the two following, the best of all others.

An

An Account of a new discovered Herb, growing wild in the Woods, exceeding all other Herbs whatsoever for supplying the Use of Hops in brewing Malt Drinks, as sent by William Ellis, Surgeon in London, to his Father at Little Gaddesden in Hertfordshire.

"SIR,

"A person acquainted me he had been ill by the
" loss of appetite some time, and being directed by a
" friend of his to the use of the following, it resto-
" red him as it did the communicator in about a
" week's time, viz by drinking half a pint of strong
" tea made from wood sage every morning fasting
" I have occasionally mentioned one of the virtues
" of wood sage as a good stomachick, and, I think, but
" little inferior to the rest of this denomination; and
" though a much despised and neglected common
" herb, yet has many other virtues, from the sancti-
" on of the celebrated John Ray, M A. late fel-
" low of the Royal Society, who in his catalogue of
" plants growing in England, gives this species of
" sage the following character
" A decoction of this herb (says he) promotes a dis-
" charge of urine, and is profitably given in the vene-
" real disease. It is particularly an excellent vulne-
" rary, either taken in potions inwardly, or outward-
" ly applied It seems to agree in virtue with the
" scordium, or, as Schroder will have it, with clary.
" It is (says he) a notable antiscorbutick ——— This
" is an exact translation from the Latin, and I should
" think enough upon the whole to supplant the use of
" the hop, particularly in a dear season, especially as
" it is so easily attained, growing plentifully in most
" woods or hedges, on dry rising grounds But I be-
" lieve its use in brewing is a secret only in our breasts,
" since the ingenious physician Dr Strother from
" whom I obtained it is since dead And I think he
" told me the brewers were ignorant of this fine bit-
" ter."

The next best Vegetable for supplying the Hop is Daucus Seed, or the Seed of the Wild Carrot.

This grows wild in our Chiltern dry country. Its seedy head is like that of the garden carrot, and is ripe in August. Its virtues are hot and dry in the third degree, chiefly used for obstructions in the liver and spleen, ureters, coughs, asthmas, cholick, pleurisies, and stranguries. It expels wind, and helps to stop lasks and overcomes poison ——— A person at Whitchurch in Bucks boiled a handful of yarrow with as much daucus seed in water, then put the water over a bushel of malt, and drank it without boiling ——— This he said strengthened his bowels, and helped him to retain his water, which otherwise would run from him. Some therefore have brewed daucus ale, and sold it for a higher price than ordinary.

But when the wild carrot seed is to supply the use of hops, it should be just bruised and tied up loosely in linen, and boiled only a quarter of an hour in the wort. A large handful of this seed is enough for a kilderkin of ale. If for long keeping, some hops must be added.

The best way to extract the purest and finest Part or Spirit of Herbs.

Formerly doctors of physick used to direct decoction or boiling of herbs to get out their virtue. But of late years they have learned more wit, and directed to do it by infusion only; else if herbs or flowers are boiled long, it will cause their finest parts or spirits to fly off, and the liquor become impregnated with an ill-tasted, earthy, austere and unwholesome quality ———

N. B. All herbs to be made use of in brewing should be carefully gathered in a dry day, in their greatest perfection and height of sap, and kept dryed in the shade in paper bags for this purpose in a dry condition.

How curious a certain Lord in the North of England is in having his Malt dryed leisurely sweet.

This Lord is so curiously nice in having his malt dryed of a pale colour, and in the highest degree of perfection of sweetness, that he obliged his maltman to be drying a kiln of it two days and two nights, by the fewel of his pit-coal charked or coaked, and this on a kiln made with bricks or tiles full of large holes at bottom, but in its upper part no bigger than large pin holes, and this by so moderate a degree of heat, that it is near a sun's heat, which gives the malt a crisp bite and pale colour——————This malt kiln they clean and clear by picking its holes with a nail, but chiefly by the sweep of a birch broom. He thus has eighteen bushels dryed at a time, and indeed he is very right in so doing.

How to boil Wort in an open Copper without wasting it.

Begin to boil your wort with as much violence as you can, and as it boils, put now and then some warm water into the copper, but so as not to stop the boiling. This will make the wort break the sooner into large particles, especially if at first you put in a spoonful of salt to half a hogshead of wort. Thus you may boil one or two hours without wasting, for it is only the additional watery part that flies off in vapour or steam, and not the wort, for the wort is an oily balsamic body, therefore though the water is thus added to it, yet the wort will have its due cure in boiling, as much as if no water was added to it. And to know if you have not lessened your quantity of wort in thus boiling, it may be proved by fixing a piece of cork about two or three inches in breadth at the end of a stick on which it must slide, and when you would know it, put the stick to the bottom of the vessel and slide the cork to touch the surface, which afterwards may be your gage —————— Or you may make a scratch on the inside of the copper, at the height the

wort

wort was at when the water was firſt put into the copper

The Earl of Denbigh's Way to brew with whole Malt Kernels.

He had boiling water poured on his whole malt when it was in the maſh-tub, and after he had thoroughly wetted them, he had one buſhel put over eight, as a capping or cover to keep in the ſteam or ſpirit of the malt. Thus he let his hot water and malt lie four hours very cloſely covered before it run off. And for making a ſecond wort, he had another parcel of boiling water put over the malt, and maſhed it, as he did the firſt time. And when this had likewiſe remained four hours undiſturbed, the wort was drawn off in a tranſparent fineneſs ——— Both theſe worts were boiled with freſh hops, and worked with yeaſt as uſual ——— Thus this curious Lord had the fineſt of malt drink, becauſe by this method he got the firſt and beſt ſpirits out of the malt, free of that foulneſs which generally attends the brewing of ground malt. He had alſo the paleſt of malt as well as the ſweeteſt, by reaſon he had it dryed with charcoal made with the largeſt ſtalks of furze, which is allowed to make the very beſt of charcoal.

To brew Welch Ale.

Having boiled your water very well with bran in it, put it into a little maſh-tub, with three or four pecks of ground malt, ſtir it well, then put it up ſo ſtirred into a bigger maſh-tub, and thus proceed till all your malt is ſo ſerved, let it ſtand covered three or four hours, and then run it off in as ſmall a ſtream as you can, ſprinkling the top of your malt once in three or four minutes with boiling water; by ſo doing you will not diſturb the ſediment, and may have a drink as ſtrong or ſmall as you pleaſe ——— The reſt of the brewing muſt be done in the uſual way.

A new Method of brewing a table Beer, by boiling Malt and Hops together.

This is done with ground malt, without letting it stand in a tub to be mashed. Suppofing your copper holds half a hogshead, and only a bushel of malt is to be made use of for making a barrel or thirty-six gallons of table small beer. In the first place over-night, put half the malt into a tub with cold water, here to remain till next morning. Do the same by putting the other half bushel to cold water in the copper, here also to remain soaking all night. Next morning put into the copper a bag of hops, and boil the malt and hops very swiftly for half an hour or more, when you are to strain the liquor through a hair sieve into your cooling tubs. This done boil the other half bushel of malt with a bag of fresh hops, in the same manner you did the first,———work and ferment both worts together, and the brewing is finished.

The advantage of brewing small beer thus, is this. ———You have the small beer made with the first and best spirit of the malt and hops, free of that phlegmatick earthy quality which small beer is impregnated with, when brewed from grains after strong beer. Besides which, you thus brew small beer in a quick and cheap manner; for by this contrivance of soaking the malt a whole night before it is brewed, the virtue is the easier extracted.

Of preparing Backs or Coolers

These should be perfectly clean and sweet, for on this and laying your worts shallow in them to cool quickly, depends the drink's retaining a sound body, and a pleasant durable taste. For the greater assurance of which, some have their coolers lined with a thin milled lead, being of a sweeter and cooler nature than wood, and as there is no joint in the lead, are much easier cleaned; for this reason it is that dairies of late are furnished with leaden square utensils for keeping their milk longer sweet, and for cleaning them with

the

the less trouble. A finger's depth of wort is safer than a greater depth, for preventing that nasty unwholesome disease in drink called by the London brewer—*fox'd*,—which happens by unclean coolers, or by laying worts too thick in them; and when this is the case, such fox'd drink will not only taste unpleasant, but will also grow soon stale, or sour, and perhaps become ropy. And what adds to this evil is, that such tainted coolers are not easily recovered ———— The remedy is, just to wet their bottoms and side, and cast slacked stone lime over them, but bay salt will answer better; let it lie thus a day, or a day and night, then to wash all clean with scalding water, thus the lime or salt will enter into the joints and crevices of the wood, and destroy the taint beyond any other thing.

The Method of working or fermenting Drink in an open Tun or Tub.

This is also a very material article in brewing, for without a right judgment in working wort, the whole brewing may be spoiled; therefore in summer let your wort be near cold before you put your yeast to it, in winter, a little more than blood warm. But for the safer and surer doing this———— Take two or three quarts of the wort, and put some yeast to it, in an earthen pot or pan, and when it has well fermented here, stir the same into the whole body of the wort, but be sure not to beat or whisk the yeast in, as the present custom is with too many of the London and country brewers, although it is so very injurious to the drinker's health, that it is a pity there is not a law to restrain that abominable practice, for by beating the yeast in, it flattens and suffocates the fine penetrating virtues of the drink, by which it is impregnated with a strong fulsome sweetness, that too many of the ignorant people admire, and the more, as such yeast-beaten ale or beer appears extraordinary fine in a glass, which it seldom fails to do, as yeast is the heavier body than the wort, and also for its potent intoxicating quality, *improving Malt Liquors.*

quality, which gives them to believe it is the mere strength of the malt, and the more nourishing, when indeed such yeasty liquor fails not to fur, foul and obstruct the stomach and passages sending up dark dulling fumes and vapours into the head, and also generates a hard gritty quality in people's blood, for yeast is an acid and breeds scurvy, gravel and stone. Therefore its evil consequences ought the more to be avoided, for it is surely a poisonous ingredient, as is proved by its killing swine, which has happened to some, by giving them the grounds of barrels. It is likewise said that a yeasted toast, being given to a hungry dog, swelled and poisoned him. The same to a human body, but in a slower degree, by tipling of such yeast-beaten ale or strong butt beer. But what careth the brewer, or the publican, since the first, by beating in the yeast a week together in winter, saves a bushel or two of malt in eight, and the last, by selling it at a fine ale price. I therefore advise all brewers, not to stir or beat their yeast into their working drink above once, but to tun or barrel it when it has worked into a strong yeasty curled head, ———— as to the working or fermenting small beer it is a general rule with the great common London brewer, especially in summer time when it has worked into a creamy head, to tun it directly, for if small beer has work'd much, it will lose its spirits sooner than stronger beer

The Method of working or fermenting Ale, or Strong Beer, in the Barrel.

This is much practised in some parts of the West country. They first put some yeast and wort together in a pail, and when it has fermented well, they put it into the barrel; and upon this, they pour in their strong raw wort. till they fill the vessel near full. Here they let it work thoroughly at first, else it would be sputtering for some time. If it works too much, their remedy is to draw some out, and fill up with cold raw wort to check it. This done, if it is for keeping, they don't rack it off ———— Thus they work

work their butt beer, for preventing (as they say) too much of the spirit of the drink flying off in the fermentation, which in an open tun or tub, it is very apt the more to do ———— If they do this in winter, they observe to put a pail full of scalding water first into the cask, to warm and better prepare it to forward the working of the whole drink

To make Grounds of Barrels supply the Want of Yeast

In case you have a cask that has fresh grounds in it, and you are in want of yeast, heat a pail full of your raw wort, scalding hot, and put it directly into such a cask, stirring it well about. Then at an hour's end, pour into your cask all your raw wort, to the warm wort first put in, and as this has well fermented, it will ferment and work all the rest

To ferment and work drink without Yeast.

Take whites of eggs, and soundly beat them; then mix flour, salt, and some coarse sugar; this mix well with the warm wort, and it will work it without yeast

To preserve Yeast some time sweet.

When your yeast is plenty, take a quart of it, and stir and work it well with a whisk, till it comes thinish, then get a large wooden bowl, platter, or tub, clean and dry, and with a soft brush, besmear the yeast all over the bottom and sides of it, and let it dry on the same ———— Or put a new birch broom into the yeast as it is working in the tun or tub, and dry the yeast on it, which keep in a dry place till wanted, or pour off the thin part, and reserve the thick part, dry the same in the air, or by a fire, mix salt with it, and keep it in rolls, in a dry place, or put yeast into a wide mouth'd bottle, well corked, and lay it in a pond or river, or cool cellar.

To make bitter Yeaſt ſweet.

Some put long bran into a linen cloth, and upon this the bitter yeaſt, which mixing together in the cloth, they pour on hot water, ſtirring till the yeaſty part is waſhed out of the bran ———— Others pour cold water on the yeaſt in a pan, and when all is well ſettled, ſo that the water appears clear, they pour it off from the yeaſt, repeating it until the bitterneſs is gone off in the water ———— This is the common way of curing yeaſt, which is weakened by this proceſs.

To recover the working of Drink, when it is too backward

This is done by an iron inſtrument ; in this are put embers or live coals, or the heater of a ſmoothing box-iron, and by its handle dip it into the drink, and preſently take it out, if there be occaſion.———— this is done for more than one reaſon, firſt for heating the cold wort, and cauſing it to ferment ; ſecondly, it helps to take off the rawneſs of the malt, when it is not thoroughly dryed, and thereby mellows and improves the drink.———— Others will fill a large ſtone bottle with ſcalding water, and by letting it lye well corked in the drink, it will heat and forward its working, which is much better than heating wort over a fire, and adding it to the reſt

To make amber Malt produce a pale Ale or Beer.

Put wheat flour, or ſmall bran over your maſh ;—— or boil pale honey in the wort

To make Strong Drink Somewhat Stronger.

A publican does this that brews his own drink, ſaying, he can make ſtronger drink from the ſame malt, than others do who are ignorant of the method. ———— Inſtead of waſhing his ſtrong beer caſks in ſcalding water, as the common way is, he only rinces them with cold water, for his notion is, that if ſcalding water is used, it scalds out the strength of the last strong drink.

Two excellent Accounts of Brewing Pale Beer, as practised in Kent.

I. A certain wine cooper, at Rochester, his method of brewing four bushels of pale-malt, of which he made half an hogshead of strong beer, and the like quantity of small.———He took his liquor just before it boiled, and mashed two bushels of the malt and made three worts, which he put all together in his copper, brought it into a boiling pitch, and mashed the other two bushels with it, letting it run off upon two pounds of fine hops a little rubbed between the hands, then into the copper with them, and boiled only till the hops sunk, which was about a quarter of an hour———work'd it cool, freed it as much as may be from the lees or grofs part, and in a few months enjoyed an excellent liquor.

All liquors are best when most freed from their lee, and therefore keeping beers should be racked two or three times as well as wines, and managed in the same manner i e when they are racked to have the following composition put into them———He puts about an ounce of fine white isinglass beat and cut small, into a gallon of stum, (which they sell at most cyder merchants for two shillings per gallon) when dissolved it will be like a thick syrup—of which, when strained, he used to put three pints into a butt of beer (or wine) when racked off, stirring it well with a broom or mop-stick, slit into four at the lower end.

This wine forcing, he says, he has found to be far better for fining and preserving malt liquors than the common way, and very much improves the beer——— He racks his beer as soon as he finds it pretty fine, and lets the bung be out a few hours before, which contributes to its fining,———lets it stand about a month or two, then racks again, then in about three or four months after, repeats the same for the last time; always observing to put in the forcing immediately after racking.———Nine

―――Nine or ten months, he says, is old enough for beer, and that this is right management, to have a fine, mellow, agreeable and well-tasted malt liquor, not inferior to our foreign wine, and 'tis the defect of it that causes so much bad foul stuff among us, which very often (in the stale beers) becomes a third part vinegar, by letting them stand upon their lee.

―――Their wines, he says, would be as bad, was it not for this management or cooperage, and was it not absolutely necessary, why should so many hundreds of them be employed?

As to the common objection against racking, and the use of isinglass, that it flats and subjects the beer to decay, he says it is true, it will flat at first, and so does wines, but provided the drink has a good body, no one by this management need fear its becoming both brisk and fine in a little time.

He uses two instruments, which are very necessary in racking, one by way of a large gimblet, which takes a piece of wood out at once, to let in a large brass cock ――――The other is to tilt steadily and gradually the large vessel as it lies upon its side or bouge on the filling.

He strains his bottoms both of wine and beer, thro' a sort of cloth called drill, which is far better than flannel, because this last is only, the other not, and it will run thro' much sooner and as fine by returning it once or twice.

II Mr Weller, at the Castle at Ashford in Kent, his method of brewing nine hogsheads of strong pale beer, which he sold for four pence a quart, and two hogsheads of small ――He had the thinnest, lightest and best pale beer in Kent, in the year 1738.

He used for his pale malt that which was dryed with oak and Welch coal mixed――as to his brown, it was straw dryed.

He brewed three days together, and wetted about thirty bushels of malt each time――――The first day, he put four hogsheads of liquor (though it was from a pump yet it lathered well) just before it boiled upon

upon the thirty bushels, through a trunk set upon a false bottom full of holes (allowing a third for waste) mashed and let it stand only two hours, then spent away by a stream about the bigness of a tobacco pipe bowl (which took about half an hour in running off) then pump'd up this first wort into the copper, and put five pounds of hops (not rubbed) into it, and boiled two hours or an hour and half at least,————strained his hops through a basket, which he hoisted up with a pulley, over his cooling bag to strain————then directly away with them into the copper to the second wort (which was made by putting three hogsheads or hardly so much upon the same goods, and let stand the same time) he boiled this two or three hours, by which time, the first wort was cooled, and let this down fine into the working tun————and his second wort in its stead————Then put up three hogsheads of cold liquor over the same goods, and let it stand an hour or an hour and half, then drew it off and put it into the copper, made it boil and threw the basket of hops to lie in it all night;————second day————in the morning he boiled it again, and returned it on 27 bushels of fresh malt (allowing three bushels for the return) heating another copper full of liquor, of which he put over the same goods one hogshead to compleat his mash, and for his second wort, &c as he did the day before;————third day————he proceeded as before————And for small beer at last, he did as for the returned worts, only making what quantity he pleased, and using as many of the last hops as he thought fit

He let the second worts lye in the coolers all night, and passed them down the next morning to the first, which he had set to work the night before as soon as ever it was cool enough.

He cleansed every other day, by a leaden pipe (fixed to the bottom of his working tun) which passed all under ground into his vessels in the cellar, by the help of three leathern pipes with brass screws to fix to the end of them

It

It worked in the veffels for three days, and he kept filling them up with what worked out, for he faid, 'tis the beft that works out

His copper held three hogfheads,————and he let off his wort fo fine from his mafh-tun, that one might read a pretty large print, looking through a glafs of it————He had put two cooling-bags, and a cock or arm to his copper————He ftrained his fettlings from the coolers through a canvas, becaufe it ftrains more expeditioufly, and wafheth better than flannel

Here they lay their under-backs and leaden pipes with an earth called duff, dug two miles from hence at a place called Kennington Lees, which, they fay, will preferve them for an hundred years or more.

H————den, Efq, has at his country-feat one of the beft furnifhed cellars of beer in the kingdom————He puts hops for the wort to run on, and then puts wort and them into the copper, and boils only five minutes, and while it is boiling a man ftrews falt over the boiling wort and hops, which will caufe the hops to fink prefently; and then they ftrain off the wort————He barrels it two years, and keeps it in bottles feveral more

To mellow and improve Beer brewed from under-dryed Malt

Ale or beer brewed from raw or under-dryed malt cannot be a pleafant wholefome liquor, no more than flefh can make good broth or foup, if but half or three quarters boiled; yet as bad as this ill property is to malt and drink brewed from it, it reigns more now than ever, for there is little malt dryed leifurely and in its full time, fo as to make right brewings of good ale or beer, becaufe the malfter grudges fewel, labour and time,————therefore it is a pity there is not a law made to oblige malfters to give their malt its due time of drying on the kiln————However, to fupply this defect in fome meafure, I here propofe what is in practice by fome, viz

The first way to cure the ill effects of raw dryed malt ———— It is done by an iron, full of very small holes, like those in a colander, and in shape of a warming-pan, wherein live coals or embers are to be put for quenching them in the wort; and if it is thought fit, after the first pan of coals becomes cold, more live ones may be put into it. Besides which, in case ale or beer is backward in working, (as I have before observed) by this the same may be presently warmed, so as to make it vigorously ferment and work ———— A second way is, to make use of a burnt billet of beech-wood, for beech is the properest wood of all others for this purpose; and when the billet is so burnt as to be all on fire, and fully divested of smoak, dip it into the wort as it is boiling in the copper, and it will mellow and help to fine the drink, and make it have a brisk taste. ———— A third way is, to roast and parch wheat kernels till they are black, and boil them in the wort, and it will much help to cure the rawness of malt, far better than by putting raw wheat kernels into a barrel of ale or beer.

Brewing strong October Beer without boiling the Wort or Hops

A certain man at Froome in Somersetshire, who used to brew for gentlemen, assured me he never boiled the wort (made from the best pale malt, that when broke one might as it were chalk with it) and always infused his hops in boiling water, which was afterwards added to the wort and worked together, and made excellent drink

To fine and preserve Beer.

Cut a piece round a loaf and break it in bits exceeding hard, and put them with a pint of wheat into a hide-kin of October beer, to lay a year

Another way ———— Some of the *London* dealers in *Dorchester* beer, I am credibly informed, when they find a large cask or hogshead of this drink become sour-

improving Malt Liquors 219

ish or upon the decay, remedy it by cutting a hot well-baked two-penny loaf in pieces and putting it therein, if a little foul or stale, they add half a pint of stum at the same time, and stir it well with a slit broomstick.

Another ———— A certain topping brewer and innkeeper in the country, when he finds his pale beer inclining to turn eager, ———— to preserve it in a sound mellow state, puts fresh hops into a bag, with a chalkstone in the bottom, and sinks it in the beer, and it will improve it and keep it good a long time

To fine half an hogshead of small new Ale

Take a handful of hops that have been boiled in a first wort and dryed, a large lump of loaf sugar, oyster-shell powder, and the stems of tobacco pipes that have been used and burnt again and powdered, of each four ounces, mix these ingredients, and put them into a cask when the ale has done working, stirring the whole well about with a staff, ———— bung down directly, and in 12 or 14 hours it will bear a glass as well as drink of six months old ———— These ingredients will not only fine drink, but also preserve it good and make it more wholesome than ordinary; the oyster-shells should be those calcined or bleached by the sun, or next best, those freed from their dirt or grit, and baked white in a slack oven

To recover pricked beer

In half an hogshead put two quarts of wheat or one quart of horse-beans whole all loose; put in also half a pound of hops in a very thin bag with a weight, (a chalk-stone is best to sink them) this will sometimes cause a small fermentation, and if taken in time, will have the desired effect

To lessen Beer fermenting in the Tun

Sprinkle cold water over it

To stop fermenting too much in the barrel.

Mix four ounces of sugar with a handful of salt, and put it in

To give pale Ale a pleasant Gout, and make it headier.

A certain *London* common brewer used to boil coriander seed in it, and it took mightily till discovered

To give brown Beer a deeper colour

There are many ways of doing it, but if it is done by boiling in the wort a little red saunders or some madder root in gross powder, if not too much, it will answer, give it no disagreeable relish, and is very wholesome

New Way of Bunging a Barrel.

First put on a piece of linen cloth, and then brown paper pasted with yeast or otherwise on that,——— then put sand mixt with brine over all ———This is called the best of bunging

Of the Nature of Malts

Malts are chiefly made good or bad, according to the fewel they are dryed with, and the time allowed for the same, &c In most parts of the west their malts are so stenched with the smoak of wood, with which they are dryed, that no stranger can endure it, though the inhabitants who are familiarized to it, can swallow the liquor so impregnated with seeming pleasure But the *London* common brewer by his art manages his wood-dryed malt so well that the tang of it is not perceived in his porter-beer, with which and a mixture of pale-malt he brews it, the slack drying rawness of the last overcoming the dryed burnt tang of the first Thus their brown malt is drying or rather

scorching

scorching an hour and half, and their pale perhaps, eight hours. Whereas to dry a brown malt in a right degree, it should have eight hours; amber malt twelve, and pale malt four and twenty at least drying, on a kiln. But (says the brewer) such leisurely dryed malt will cost us too much, to return a sufficient profit. Therefore I advise all, to have a special regard to the malt they brew with——The best malt is dried with wheat straw, or with coak, or with Welch coal,——coak gives a fine coat to malt, else the more knowing will not approve of it.

To know good from bad malt

Bite the malt kernel across in the middle of it or at both ends, and if it tasteth mellow and sweet, has a plump body, breaks softish, is full of flour all its length, smells well, and has a thin skin, it is then a good sort——You may also know good from bad malt, by putting some into a glass of water, that which swims is right, but that which sinks is steely, and not true malt——Avoid also making use of under-dried, or what we call raw-dried malt, which gives drink a maukish taste, and disagreeable unwholesome quality——I had much rather drink beer or ale brewed from brown too high-dryed malt, by a sweet fewel, than than that brewed from a raw-dryed malt, tho' of a tempting pale colour

Waters, their Nature for brewing.

Soft water, or water that will easily lather, with soap, agrees best with brown malt, and amber malt, but for pale malt, spring hard water is best——I have known black-horse pond made use of, to brew October strong beer, and it has proved excellent, but then some salt should be boiled in it to raise a scum, which should be carefully taken off——Well hard water is softened by exposing it some time to the air, or infusing a bag of wood ashes in it

Of Wort breaking in the Copper.

This is a material point in brewing to observe — If wort is under or over-boiled, they are extreams; to boil it to a true crisis, boil it till it breaks into particles as big as grains of wheat, then it is just right to take out of the copper, for by this the drink will work well in the tun, and fine well in the barrel —— If under-boiled it will be raw tasted, if over-boiled it will be thicker bodied, and in neither case become so fine, pleasant and wholesome, as when the wort is finely broken in the copper —— If the second water or wort stands too long on the malt, it will be of a greyish colour, and never break in boiling —— The brisker wort boils, the sooner it will break, for if wort boils too long, it becomes (as I before observed) thicker bodied, and a heavier drink, not brisk, because by too long boiling, the mucilaginous parts are the more predominant and fixed.

How to make Wort break the sooner.

When wort and hops have boiled a little, dissolve half a pint of salt in some water, and put it into your barrel or hogshead copper, and it will make it break the sooner, give the drink a good relish, keep it sound the longer, and cause it to fine the sooner. Or take about half an ounce of true salt of tartar (which at the *London* chemists is sold for two-pence an ounce) and mix it well with your hops that are to be boiled in the wort, and it will help to break and fine it, by seperating the foul particles and throwing them down sooner, than in the common way. Some, instead of salt of tartar, rub their hops with common salt, but that is not near so good as the other. Others put in a pound of common salt into a hogshead of wort just before it boils, to break it quickly into curds, and save much boiling.

To lay Wort thin

It should never be laid to cool thicker than a finger's length deep ——— It is the laying the wort thick, that causes many thousand barrels of drink to be foxed

To clean the inside of a foul cask

Take a stick about the bigness of a broom handle, eighteen inches more or less in length, cut notches at its end, for tying a cloth the faster about it, with this, scrub and rub the inside of the cask very clean, till the fur and slime is entirely got off. If a man's hand will not enter, a boy's will, and thus do it with either cold or scalding water. Some fasten a piece of an old birch broom to the end of a stick, and make it answer this purpose

How to sweeten a stinking cask, by lime

This is known to be a good sweet way, when a cask is not thoroughly tainted ——— First, fill it up with boiling water, and immediately put the lime-stones in, and every now and then, and they will raise and continue the ebullition

Another more effectual way to sweeten a stinking cask by fire.

This is done by the fire of wheat straw ——— In the southams of *Devonshire*, where they make abundance of cyder, they take out one of the heads of a hogshead, and setting it upright, after it is thoroughly cleaned, they burn wheat straw in it, a little at a time, and so on for perhaps a quarter of an hour ——— But this position, I take not to be so good as I have practiced, and that is, when I have the head taken out, I lay the hogshead on the ground sideways, and burn wheat straw in it, a little at a time, for a quarter of an hour, and in burning it, I turn the cask now and then, till the heat of the fire has penetrated through the staves of the cask. Thus the remaining head in the

the cask, is not so liable to damage by the fire as when the cask stands upright. When the cask is thus fired, scald it well with boiling water, to discharge the smoak of the straw.

To strengthen, relish, fine, and preserve Ale or Beer.

First Receipt.———Mix a pint of wheat flour with two pounds of bruised raisins, and two pounds of melasses or coarse sugar, or honey, a pint of clean brandy, a spoonful of salt, and an ounce of powder'd ginger.———Make this into balls, and put them into a hogshead of strong beer.

Second Receipt.———Boil two ounces of isinglass, with three pounds of hops, in two gallons of strong drink, when cold, strain and stir into a hogshead of strong ale or beer.

Third Receipt.———*For keeping pale beer.* Take the finest bean flour, wheat flour, and powder of calcin'd oyster-shells. Mix these with whites of eggs, brandy and honey, into a moist paste. Put it into one or more coarse bags, with a stone in the bottom, letting them hang by a string.———Put this into a cask as soon as the drink has done working, when it is about nine months old, it will be very fine—then you may bottle it with a horse bean in each bottle; let it stand as long in the bottles, and it will mantle and drink very soft and agreeable.

Fourth Receipt.———Some break six sea-biscuits, and putting them into a bag with hops, let it lye in a cask of strong beer,—this will keep the beer fresh, and give it a fine flavour.

Fifth Receipt.———Others put chalk into a bag, with hops, for the same purpose.

Sixth Receipt.———Some put lime stones into a cask of ale or beer; but then it should be a lime made with soft chalk, not with the hurlucky for-

If such lime is thus used, it will cause such an effervescency, or struggling of the small particles of the liquor, that when it is over, the liquor will become fine in twenty-four hours.

Seventh Receipt ———— Boil three pounds of honey with two pounds of hops, of the palest sort, a quarter of an hour; when cold, stir all well in a barrel, or hogshead of rack'd or unrack'd pale beer.

Eighth Receipt ———— As practised at *Canterbury* in *Kent* ———— Here they boil isinglass and coarse sugar together in small-beer. When cold, they mix some river sand with it, first washed clean; for if they were to make use of dry sand, it would in summer time cause the drink to fret and fume out of the bung-hole of an upright standing cask; and so careful are they here to prevent this evil in their butt-beers, that in putting this their fining, they leave the peg loose in the head of the butt, for part of the summer, for fear of damage.

Ninth way ———— In the *West* country they use the less hops at first, when they boil their wort, in order to use the more afterwards; for here they boil two pounds of hops with two pounds of coarse sugar in a little water, only a quarter of an hour, and to do this in the greater perfection, they draw off their new worked beer after it has stood in the working vat a week, as fine as they can, and then putting it into the hogshead, they stir in the hops and sugar, to feed and fine the drink for long keeping ———— Or, if the beer is already casked, it may be rack'd off into another cask, for leaving all the sediment behind, then adding the hops and sugared liquor, and it will thus fine and preserve it. Thus, if beer is in this manner managed, it will appear fine in a glass at a week's end, even beyond what isinglass can do, being a very wholesome durable finer, pleasing most palates; and it is well known, and practised by some of the most acute brewers.

To stop a leak in a cask as it stands in its place.

To do this, mix wheat flour, or flour of brimstone with the white of an egg, mix it a little warm till incorporated.

Second Way.

Mix and work tallow with powdered chalk, or wheat flour, and apply it.

A third Way.

But where a cask is empty, mix rosin with pitch, by melting them together, and run it thus melted on the leak ——— This and that above, will stop a leak in cold liquor, but not in hot.

A fourth Receipt, to stop a leak, so that scalding water has no power to overcome it.

Melt and apply brimstone alone.

To refine Beer, Ale, Cyder or Wine ——— A Hogshead.

1. Take two ounces of the best and clearest isinglass, strip it, and put it soaking in a quart of the same liquor you want to refine; beat it up two or three times a day with a whisk, and put fresh liquor to it as it thickens, and it will be all dissolved, and fit for use in twenty-four hours.

Draw off one third part of the cask you want to refine, and put it into a tub you must have ready for that purpose, then put into the cask the above preparation, with a quarter of an ounce of pearl ashes, one ounce of true salt of tartar, and one ounce of alum burnt and powdered, mix these well in the cask with a rummager, then fill up the casks, and it will fine and be fit to draw in less than three days.

Another

Another excellent Receipt to refine Beer, Cyder, and Wine, which will also recover it, if upon the turn, or turned quite sour ——For a Hogshead.

II. Take the whites of twelve eggs, with their shells, one ounce of salt of tartar, half an ounce of pearl ashes, and one pennyworth of grains of paradise bruised; mix these with as much of the powder or shavings of chalk, as will make it of the consistence of paste, roll it into small balls, and put them into beer, cyder, or wine, and they will take off the sharp particles, and make it fine, mild and pleasant in less than a week.

III. If beer or ale be flat and want more hops, boil a pound or two of the best hops (as you see occasion) in two gallons of new wort, strain it off, and work it with yeast, then put it into the cask with either of the above preparations.

This last in *Dorsetshire* is called vamping of beer.

** These three last mentioned receipts only, to some persons, are worth scores of pounds, as they will assuredly answer their character in almost all drinkable liquors, except the spirituous sort, and that for a trifling charge, and are good against the scurvy and gravel.—Nor should any hogshead of beer, wine or cyder be kept without these ingredients in it, as they give the liquor a transparent fineness, and a pleasant taste, make it more wholesome, and surely preserve it from staleing.

To recover stale Beer.

Draw it off into another cask, and put whole malt and fresh hops into it ——The hops first, just soaked in warm water, or better, if in a little of the same beer.

The best way of brewing.

Is never to mash but once, and lade boiling water over the rest till you get your due quantity; and this is justly accounted the best way of private brewing.

To fine and preserve Beer

Put treacle into a barrel of beer, with two bags of whole malt. Salt and ginger together do good service to malt drink.

To fine and preserve Butt Beer, designed for keeping long

Some have put into a butt of it, one pound of quick lime, and four pounds of lean beef.

To preserve Hoops

Mix powdered whiting with painters linseed oil, and brush it over wooden or iron hoops as a paint.

The best way to make Wormwood Ale or Purl

As there are many persons who chuse, in cold weather to drink a draught of this warm in a morning, I shall here direct them two ways of doing it in the greatest perfection——The first is to take the tops of Roman wormwood, gathered in its prime, and dried the preceding summer, a little fresh horse-radish root, cut in thin slices, and rather less of enula campana root, with some of the yellow rind of Seville oranges, dry and cut small,—as much of these as you chuse, to have the drink more or less imbittered—— Put all these into a stone or earthen jug or jar, mixed with a little true salt of tartar, and thereon pour as much boiling wort, (when boiled enough, such as that before mentioned, brewed with malt and melasses, is very suitable) sufficient to cover it well; when cold, strain off the liquor, mix and work it with the rest of your wort,——give it five or six weeks age, and it makes excellent purl——Or you may make it by a cold infusion of the same wormwood tops, some sliced gentian root, dried Seville orange peel, and juniper-berries, bruised in either brandy or good geneva—— Two or three tea spoonfuls of this tincture made strong, in a pint of warm mild ale, will also make the best of purl, abundantly pleasanter, and much more wholesome, than that commonly sold in *London*, made with their fulsome yeast-beaten twopenny

F I N I S.

INDEX.

A

Admirable Plum, to preserve green, 25
Alembic, how to distil with it, 158
Almond Butter, with Milk, 52 Butter Jelly, ib
Cakes, 84 Butter, 181 Cream, 56 Another,
ib Cream very rich, called Steeple Cream, 133
Another, 58 Custard, 59 Flummery, 61
Almonds, to preserve green, 31 To parch, 32 To
make of Chocolate, ib To preserve dry, 33.
Cakes for Figures, 34 A fine one, 187 Gingerbread, brown, 88 A second, ib Milk for a Wash, 190
Amber Plumbs, to preserve green, 23 To preserve yellow, 26
Angelica, to preserve in Knots, 15 To dry it, ibid.
To preserve in Sticks, ibid Paste, 16 Tarts, 132.
To candy, 191 Water Compound, 166 Single, 170
Anniseed Water, 120 Biscuits, 132
Antiscorbutic Water, 167
Apples, Jelly of 49 Apples and Pears to dry, 13.
Black Caps of, ibid To preserve, red, 137
Apricots, to preserve green, 17 To put up in Jelly, 18 To preserve whole, ib Chips, 19 In Jellies, 20 Paste, ib Clear Cakes, ib Jam, 21.
Pears and Plumbs, to candy, 37 Jumbles, 71.
Wine, 114
Aqua Mirabilis, 170
Artificial Fruit, 90
Artichoaks, to dry red, 137
Arquebusade-Water, 171
Arms, how to be kept from rust, 188.

INDEX

B

Balm water, 99
Balsam syrup, 125
Barberries, to preserve, 40. To dry, ib
Barley syrup, 125.
Bay Salt, oil of, 93
Bean, or Almond Bread, 70 Cakes, 85
Beer, to make it fine, 119
Beet Roots, to preserve, 136
Bergamot water, 172
Bills of Fare for Deserts, 140 to 150
Benjamin, Oil of, 93
Beauty water, 173
Birch Wine, 115 As made in Sussex, 117
Biscuits Ratafia, 73 Or Sugar, a cheap sort, 74.
    Savoy, ib A second, ib Lemon, ib Hard, 75
    French, iced, 76. Naples, ib Orange, ib An-
    niseed, 132 Nun's, 135 French, 189
Bitters, 105 Bitter Wine, 115
Blackberry wine, 185
Black Cherry Water Cordial, 130 Wine, 118
    Water for Children, 103
Black Caps, the best way, 134.
Blanched Cream, 59
Bloomage, 62
Bouquet's water, 174
Briton's Wine 109
Buckthorn, Syrup of, 124—128
Bullace, to preserve, 132
Butter, Orange, 53 Fairy, ib

C

Cakes, Orange, 7 Lemon, 8. White Pear Plumb,
    27 Orange clear, 9 Cheese, *see* Cheese Cakes,
    &c Rich Great, 77 Plumb, ib Icing for,
    78—79 Rich Plumb, ib Ordinary ditto, 80
    Pound Seed, ib Another, ib Rich Seed, ib
    Little Currants and Seeds, 81 Liquorice, ib
    Nun's, 82 Saffron, ib Rich Yeast, 83. Little
        Queen,

INDEX.

Queen, ib   Almond, 84   Portugal, ib   Carraway, ib   Shrewsbury, 85   Barbu.y, ib   Whetstone, ib   Bean, ib   Gum, 86   Honeycomb, ib   Lemon, ib   Lemon, Orange, and Flour, 87   Violet, ib   Wormwood, ib   Flowers, 88   Without Eggs, Sugar or Butter, ib   Pepper, 92

Calves-Foot Jelly, 48
Candied Cakes, 73
Carmes, Eau de, 169
Cardamum Water, 98, and 120
Carraway Cakes, 84   Water, 120   Spirits of, 130
Carrots to pickle, 139
Cedrat Water, 181
Cheese Cakes, 62 and 64   Of Potatoes, or Lemons, 63   Mrs Harrison's, ib   Lady Leicester's Cream, 64   Two others, ib   Orange, 65.   Rice, ib.   Ship Coat, 189
Cherry Paste, 36   Cordial, 131
Cherries, Mrs Smith's way of preserving in Jelly, 36   To preserve the French way, ib   To preserve a Cheap way, 37   To candy Mrs Smith's way, ib   To dry 34   To preserve Liquid, 35   To make Jam of, 44   Dry, how to keep 45   Brandy 105.   Morello, wine of, 114   Black, wine of, 118   Red, wine of, ib
China, how to mend, 192
Chocolate Cream, 57   Puffs, 91
Cider, See CYDER
Cinnamon water, 100—176
Citron, to make of green Mellons, 8   To preserve white, ib & 177   Water, 99.   A second, ib   Cream, 182
Civet, Essence of, 175
Clary water, 100   Spirit, 130
Clouted Cream, 59—181
Clove Water, 95   Jelly-flowers, Syrup of, 124   Jelly-flower Wine, 138
Cochineal, to preserve, 11
Codlin cream, 57   To green, 13
Cold Cream, 57
Cold Still, how to use it, 185

INDEX.

Colliflowers to pickle red, 138.
Colts-Foot, Syrup of 123
Comfits of various colours, 69
Conserves of Hips, 129 Of Red Roses, ib. Of Orange Peel, ib Of Quinces, ib
Coughs and Asthma, Syrups for 125 and 128
Cowslip Wine, 113
Cracknels, 135
Cream Snow, 52 Curd, 54 Lemon, ib Orange, ib A second sort, ib Clear Cream, 55. Yellow Lemon, ib Spanish, ib Loaf Sugar, 56 Imperial, ib. Almond, ib Another, 133 Pistachia, 57 Cold, ib Codlin, ib Rasberry, ib Chocolate, ib Almond, 58 Steeple, ib. Another, 133 Stone, 59 Clouted, ib Blanched, ib Posset, 61. Cheese, Lady Leicester's 64 Newport, Cheese of, 134 Sack like Butter, 191
Cucumbers, to preserve, 30.
Curds and Cream of Newcastle, 51 Of Rennet, ib. Of Cream, 54
Currants, to draw Jelly of, 35 In Bunches, to dry, 39 To preserve in Jelly, ib To ice, 40 Paste, ib. Jelly, 49 Black Jelly, 50 Seed Cakes, 81 Brandy, 105 Shrub, 136
Custard, Almond, 59 Orange, 60. Plain, ib Second and third, ib
Cyder, Sir John Cope's, 105 Madam Bentham's, 106 To make clear, 109. How to improve, and make it fine, 118 How to make, 186.
Cyprus Water, 175

D

Damsons to preserve, 132. Another way, 46. Wine, 114
Distilling, how to be performed by the Alembic, 158
Divine Water, 178.

INDEX.

E.

Eggs, Oil of, 136
Elder Wine, 111. Rob of, 130
Essence of Civet, 175
Eau de Carmes, 169
Eau de luce, how to make, 153.

F

Fairy Butter, 53.
Faints, the Use of, 183.
Fennel Water, 180.
Fermenting, the Use of it in distilling, 162.
Figs, to preserve green, 27. Ripe, ib. To candy, ib. And stone Fruit, how to keep sound and fit for Use all the Year, 45.
Filberts, Oil of 151
Fine, to make Beer, Wine, Cyder, &c. 118 and 119.
Flowers of all sorts, how to keep 46. To candy any sort of, 66
Floating Island, 48.
Flummery, Almond 61. Ising-glass, 62. Oatmeal, ib. Blomage ib. A pretty one, 134.
Fritters, Spanish 189.
Fruit to preserve green, 23. To keep for Tarts, 44.

G.

Garlick, to preserve, 30
Gingerbread, 89 A second, ib. Brown Almond, 88 A second sort, ib
Glass to mend, 192
Gold and Silver Lace, how to clean 193
Gooseberries, to preserve green 37 White, 38 To dry, ib. Paste, ib Clear Cakes, 39 To preserve whole, without stoning, 68 To keep the whole Year, 133

INDEX

Grapes, to preserve green, 28 In Bells to preserve in Jelly, ib In clusters to preserve with one Leaf. 29 When on the Tree, 46 When you gather them, ib Wine of, 111 and 112. To keep the whole year, 4+
Green fine, how to make 12,
Gumballs hollow Lady Leicester's 71
Gum Cakes, 86.

H.

Hard Biscuit, 75.
Hartshorn Jelly, 49
Heart-burn, Powder for 190.
Herb-water, of all sorts how to make, 104.
Hips, Conserves of, 129.
Hysterical Water, 103
Hollow Gum Balls, Lady Leicester's, 71.
Honeycomb Cakes, 86
Honey Water, 172
Hops with Gooseberries, to preserve, 67
Horse-raddish Water compound, 119 and 167.
Hungary Water, 96

I.

Jam of Rasberries, 44. Of Cherries, ib
Jamaica Pepper-Water, 165
Ice to make, 153.
Ice Cream, 91
Iced Biscuits, the French way, 76.
Icing for Cakes, 78 and 79
Jelly of Calves-feet, 48 For a Trifle, 47 Of Hartshorn, 49 Of Apples, ib Of Currants, ib. Of Black Currants, 50. Of Rasberries, ib
Jessamin Oil, 92 Water, 178
Imperial Cream, 56 Water, 168
Iron, how to be kept from Rust, 188
Ising-glass Flummery, 62.
Jumbles, of Almonds, 71 Another, ib. Of Apricots, ib.

Juniper,

INDEX.

Juniper Berries Water of, 98
Junkets, 53

K

Kidney Beans, to keep, 153.

L.

Lace, Gold and Silver Lace, how to clean, 188
Ladies Water, 178,
Lady Allen's Water, 104
Lady Hewet's, ditto, 101
Lavender Water, 97 Compound, 177.
Leaves, to green, 47
Lech, 53
Lemon, Citron, &c to preserve the Dutchefs of Cleveland's way, 6 To take out the Seeds, ib. Cakes 8 and 86. Cream, 54. Another, ib. Cream clear, 55 Cream yellow, ib Bifcuit, 74 Orange and Flour Cakes, 86 Water, 166.
Lip Salves, a fine one, 190
Liquorice Cakes, 81.
Loaf Sugar Cream, 56.
Loaves, to make white, 33.
Luting for Stills, how to make, 184.

M.

Macaroons, 75. A fecond, ib
Malmfey, Englifh 112
March Pans, 34
March-mallows, Syrup of 127 A fecond, ib
Mead, a Cheap fort, 108 Common, ib Frontiniac, 109 A fourth fort, ib
Mildew, how to take out of Linen, 138
Milk Water, 100. Punch, 116 To preferve for Ufe, 117
Mint Water, 99
Mogul Plumbs, to preferve green, 24

INDEX.

Montpellier Cordial, 172
Morella Cherry Wine, 114
Mulberries to preserve dry, 29 Syrup of, 123.
Myrrh, Oil of 93

N

Naple Biscuits, 76
Nectarines, to preserve, 21
Nettles, Syrup of, 152
Newcastle Curds and Cream, 51.
Nuns Cake, 82. Biscuit, 135.
Nutmegs, Oil of, 92 Water, 99.

O

Oatmeal Flummery, 62
Oil of Oranges, 92 Of Jessamin and Violets, ib. Of Nutmegs, ib Of Benjamin, 93 Of Storax, ib Of Myrrh, ib. Of Bay Salt, ib Eggs, 136 Of Filberts, 151 Of Paper, ib. For Family Uses, ib
Oyster Powder, 192
Oranges to preserve green, 5 To preserve with Marmalade and Lemons, 4 Seville, to preserve Liquid, also lemons, 3 Marmalade, also of Lemons, 4 Flower Paste, 9 Compote, 5 Lemon and Citron, to candy, 7 Cakes, 7 Rings and Faggots, 6 China, Zest of 7 Clear Bakes, 9 Flower Cakes, 10. Flowers, to preserve ib To put in Jelly, ib To preserve green, 5 Butter, 53 Cream, 54 Custard, 60 Leaves, 61 Cheese Cakes, 65 Flowers to candy, 67 Jumbles, 72 Biscuts, 76 Oil of, 92 Water, 95, 100, and 164 Mint Water, 104 Posset, 133 Peel, Conserves of 129 Wafers, 186. Loaves, 191

P

Palsey Water, 102 Strong Water, 121—122. The Use of, 122

Paper

INDEX.

Paper, Oil of 151
Parsley Water, Compound, 119
Paste, Puff 65 For Tarts, 66 For Pattypans, ib. For a Pasty, ib For a standing Crust, ib
Peaches to preserve whole, 21 Chips, how to preserve, 22 To put in Jelly, ib To preserve in Brandy, ib
Pears bonchretien, to make a Compote of 13. Purple to stew, 14
Pear Plumbs white, to make a clear Cake of 27. green, to keep 152
Pennyroyal Water, 99.
Pepper Cake, 92
Peppermint Water, 165—170.
Perfumed Water, 95
Perry, 106 As clear as Rock Water, 109
Piony Compound Water, 119—169
Pippins, to draw a Jelly from, 4 Knots to make, 11, For present Eating, 12 Golden, to preserve in Jelly, ib Golden, to dry, ib
Pistachia Cream, 57
Plague Water, 98, and 154
Plumbs Violet to preserve, 22 Green Amber to preserve, 23 Green Orange, to preserve 24 Green Mogul, to preserve ib Green Admirable, to preserve 25 Yellow Amber, to preserve 26 To put in Jelly, ib. Cakes, 27 and 77 Cake, a very rich one, 79. Cake, ordinary one, 80.
Pomegranate, clear Cakes, 10
Poppies, Syrup of 124 Water Cordial, 132
Portugal Cakes, 84
Potatoe, or Lemon Cheese Cakes, 63.
Powder of Oysters, 194
Powder, a sweet one for Cloaths, 188
Puff Paste, 65.

INDEX.

Q

Queen Cakes, 83.
Quinces, to preserve white, 17. White or Red, to preserve, ib. The Jelly of ib. Wine 113 & 117 Conserve of 129

R.

Rack Wine, how to 116
Raisin Wine, 110 Wine of different Flavours, 111, & 116. Wine like Port, ib Wine like Madeira, ib Spirit of 156
Rasberries, to preserve Liquid, 41 Cakes, 42 Clear Cakes, ib. & 43 Biscuits, 43 Jam, 44 Jelly, 50 Cream, 57. Brandy, 105.
Ratafia Biscuits, 73
Ratafia from Peaches, 179
Ratafia, 97. Common, ib
Red Cherry Wine, 118.
Rennet, Curds and Cream, 51.
Rhubarb Tarts, 131.
Rice Cheese Cakes, 65
Ringoe Root, to preserve, 16.
Rob of Elder, 130
Roses, Sugar of, in all sorts of Figures, 33. Cakes to burn for perfume, 95 To perfume, ib & 96. Syrup of 122 Red Conserve of, 129. Boiled, 182. Water, 176 Royal Water, 174.

S

Sage wine, 115.
Saffron Cakes, 82 Syrup of 127.
Samphire, to preserve, or dry, 41
Sans Pareille water, 173.
Sattins white how to clean, 188.
Savoy Biscuits, 74 A second sort, ib.
Scordium water, compound, 120
Seed Puffs, 73 Cakes, a Pound one, 80. Another, ib. Cake, a very rich one, ib.

Simple

INDEX.

Simple waters, how produced by Fermentation, 162. Those commonly in Use, 163
Shrewsbury Cakes, 85
Shrub, Sir John Cope's, 105 Of Currants, 136.
Silks flowered, with gold and silver in them, how to clean, 188
Snail water, 107
Snow Cream, 52 Balls, Carolina 190
Souring, to keep wine from 116.
Spanish Pap, Lady Leicester's 54 Cream 55.
Spearmint water, 165
Spirit of Clary, 130 Of Carraways, ib. Of Sugar, 156 Of Raisins, 156.
Stag's Heart water, 189
Steeple Cream, 58.
Still, how to use it, 153 When best to use, 155.
Stone Cream, 59
Storax, Oil of 93
Strawberries, &c how to keep, 46
Sugar, to clarify 1. To boil smooth, ib To blow, 2 To feather, ib To crackle, ib The Carmel, ib Little Devices of 32 Wafers, 69 Sugar of Rasberries, 72 Cakes, ib Puffs, ib. Biscuits, a cheap way, 74. Spirit of 156.
Surfeit water, 97
Sweet Marjoram, to preserve 16.
Sweetmeat Cream, 58
Sweet water, 94. Seven other sorts, 96, &c.
Syllabubs, everlasting 50. A second sort, ib A Mock one 51.
Syrup of Roses, 122 Colts-foot, 129. Of Tolu, Balsamic 123 Another sort, ib. Mulberries, ib. Poppies, 124 Violets, 124 126 Clove-jilly-flowers, 124 Buckthorn, 124 & 128 For a Cough or Asthma, 125 and 128 Another sort, ib Of Balsam, 125 Barley, ib Marsh-mallows, Another way, ib Saffron, 127 Of water Cresses, 152 Of Nettles, ib.

T.

INDEX.

Tarts of Rhubarb, 131 Of Angelica, 132.
Tolu, Syrup of 123
Treacle water, 102.
Trifle, a great one 47.
Tumblets 73 and 136.
Turnips, to pickle 138.

U.

Varnish, yellow 187. To cover Baskets, ib. &c.
Vestal water, 175.
Violets to rock and candy, 14 To candy whole, ib Plumbs to preserve, 22. Syrup of, 124 & 126 Cakes, 87 Oil of, 92. Drops, 138.
Usquebaugh, 106 French, 178.

W.

Wafers, 68—69 Sugar, ib. Right Dutch, 135
Walnuts, to preserve white, 29 To preserve Black Mrs Johnson's way, 30 To preserve with Filberts, 46 Water, 98. To keep all the Year, 15 & 139.
Water Cresses, Syrup of 152.
Wardens baked to a Compote, 14
Waters sweet, variety of 94. Orange, 95, 100 & 164 Clove, 95 Perfumed, ib Fine sweet, 96 Hungary, ib Lavender, 97 Ratafia, Surfeit, ib. & 135 Plague, 98 & 154 Walnut, ib. Cardamum, ib Nutmeg, 99 Mint, Balm, and Pennyroyal, ib Citron, ib & 177 Cinnamon, 100 & 176 Milk, ib Clary, ib Lady Hewet's, 101 Treacle, 102 Palsey, ib Hysterical, 103 Black Cherry, ib Lady Allen's, 104 Herb, ib Orange-mint, ib Wormwood, 107. Simple, ib Snail, ib Parsley, 119 Horse-raddish, 119 & 161 Piony, ib & 169. Scordium, 120 Anniseed, ib Carraway, ib. Cardamum, ib Strong Palsey, 121. Use of it, 122 Black Cherry, 130 Simple, how produced, 162 Simple, in use 163 Peppermint, 165 & 170 Spearmint, ib Of Jamaica Pepper, 165.

INDEX.

165 Of Lemon, 166 Angelica compound, 166. Wormwood, 167 Antiscorbutick, ib Imperial, 168 De Carmes, 169 Wonderful, 170 Angelica single, ib Arquebusade, or vulnerary, 171. Bergamot, 172 Montpellier, ib. Honey, ib. Sans Pareille, 173 Of Beauty, ib. Royal, 174. Bouquet, ib Cyprus, 175 Vestale, ib Rose, 176 Lavender, 177 Ladies, 178 Jessamin, ib Divine, ib. Cedrat, 181. Cordial Poppy, 182. Stag's-heart, 189.

Whetstone Cakes, 85

Whigs, 89. Light ones, 90.

Whim-whams, 51

Wine, to rack 116. To scent, and give a curious Flavour, ib To keep from souring, 116. Black Cherry, 118 Red Cherry, as made in Kent, 118. To make it fine, 119 Clove-jilly-flower, 138.

Wine Briton's, 109 Raisin, 110 Elder, 111. Raisin to give different flavours, ib. Like Red Port, ib Like Madeira, ib Grape, ib, 112 Cowslip, 113 Quinces, ib & 117 Morello Cherry, 114 Apricot, ib Damsin, ib Birch, 115 As made in Sussex, 117. Sage, 115 Bitter, ib. Blackberry, 185

Wormwood Cakes, 87 Water, 107 & 167. Simple water, 107

Y.

Yeast Cake, rich one, 83.

THE

THE INDEX TO THE New Art of Brewing.

A

ALE strong, how to be brewed without boiling Wort and Hops, 197. How to be brewed by boiling Water, Wort and Hops, 199. Stronger than usual, how to be made from a certain Quantity of Malt, 202. How to be fined, 224.

B

Backs and Coolers, how to be prepared, 209
Barley, how to have a white Colour, 195. To try if good ib.
Beer strong, or Norfolk Nog, how to brew, 200
Beer, from undried Malt, how to be improved, 217. How to be fined and preserved, 218. Brown, how to have its Colour heightened, 220. How to be relished, fined, and preserved, a variety of Methods, 224. Wine or Cyder, how to be refined, 226. Stale, how to be recovered, 227. If turned, ib.
Brewing, the best Method for a private Family, 222
Bruied Malt, how to brew with it, 196
Bunging of Barrels, a new Method, 220
Butt Beer, how to be preserved, 228

Cask.

INDEX.

C
Casks, a foul one how to be cleansed, 223 Stinking, how to be sweetened, ib When leaky, how to be stopped, 226

D
Daucus seed, its Use in the place of Hops, 206
Denbigh Earl of, his manner of brewing, 203.
Drink, how to be fermented in an open Tub, 210. in the Barrel, 211 How to be fermented with the Grounds of a Barrel, for want of Yeast, 212 How to be fermented without Yeast, ib When too backward in working, how to be forwarded, 213. How to be strengthened, ib
Double Beer, how to be brewed, 202.

F
Family Small Beer, how to be brewed, 197
Fermentation in the Tun, how to be lessened, 219. In the Barrel, 220.

H
Herbs to supply the use of Hops, 203, 205, 206.
How to extract the purest Spirit from, 206
Hops how to be preserved, 228
How to brew Family Small Beer, 197 Strong Ale, without boiling Wort or Hops, ib Strong Ale, by boiling Wort and Hops together, 199 Strong Beer, or Norfolk Nog, 200 Double Beer, 202 With whole Malt Kernels, 208 Welsh Ale, ib. Table Drink, by boiling Malt and Hops together, 209

M.
Malt and Hop Kiln, a new-invented one, 203 To dry, in a curious manner, 207 Kernels, how to brew with, 208. How to be prepared, for pale Ale 213 Its Nature, 220. How to be distinguished to advantage, 221.

O
October beer to be brewed, without boiling the Wort or Hops, 218.

P.
Pale Drink, how to be made from Malt, 213. How made in Kent, 214. How to give it a Flavour, 220

Pricked

INDEX.

Pricked Beer, how to recover, 219.

S.

Small Beer, how to brew, 197. How to be fined, 219

Stinking Casks, how to sweetened, 223

T

Table Drink to be made by boiling Malt and Hops together, 209

W.

Water, the best sort for brewing with, 221.

Welsh Ale, how to be brewed, 208

Wild Carrots, their Use, in the place of hops, 206.

Wormwood Ale the best way to make it, 228.

Wort, how to be boiled without wasting, 207. Of breaking in the Copper, its use, 222 For breaking in the Copper, how to be forwarded, ib How to be laid in the cooling Vessels, 223.

Y

Yeast the want of, how to be helped, 212 Without it, how to work Drink, ib How to be preserved, ib For want of, how to work Drink, with the Grounds of a Barrel, ib. Bitter, how to be made sweet, 213.

FINIS.

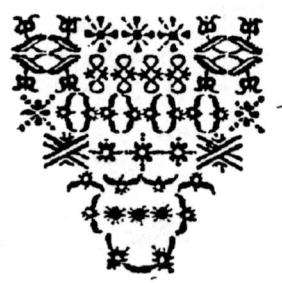

CPSIA information can be obtained at www.ICGtesting.com
Printed in the USA
LVOW111943110413

328769LV00012B/545/P